Fat to Fit Formula

Unlocking the Secrets
to Comprehensive
Weight Management

Brenda F. Dozier

Table of content

Introduction

When it comes to the never-ending goal of optimal health and well-being, the pursuit of a transforming path from fat to fit serves as a beacon of resiliency and self-discovery. Within the confines of comprehensive weight management is the key to unlocking this potential, which is contained within the human body, which is a marvel of complexity that contains the potential for deep transformation. You are cordially invited to participate in a discussion that goes beyond transient fads and shallow fixes. This is an investigation that is founded on research, enriched by experience, and personalized to the individual who is looking for a long-lasting transformation.

We have a fundamental understanding of body composition, which serves as the foundation for this experience. We go beyond the numbers that appear on a scale and explore the complexities of body fat percentage and muscle mass in order to reveal the true measures of a healthy physique. A sophisticated approach to weight control, one that acknowledges the complex structure of the human body, can be developed with the help of this basic information, which lays the platform for such an approach.

We debunk the myths surrounding the mechanisms that govern fat burning and weight regulation by delving into the science that underpins weight loss. This allows us to get to the bottom of the riddles surrounding metabolism and hormone regulation. Having acquired this information, we proceed to make a smooth transition into the domain of practical nutrition essentials, where we will create a meal plan that is well-balanced and highlight superfoods that provide the body with nourishment while also promoting sustainable weight reduction.

On the other hand, changing from being overweight to being fit is a process that goes beyond the domains of nutrition and into the territory of physical exercise. Exercise routines that are beneficial include cardiovascular activities that are meant to maximize fat burning and strength training approaches that are aimed toward the development of lean muscle mass. Our investigation into effective exercise routines was conducted. In this holistic approach, we establish a synergy between diet and exercise, acknowledging their symbiotic significance in the pursuit of a better self.

However, the mind, frequently an ignored player in the weight management symphony, takes center stage as we delve into the realms of mental wellness. The psychology of weight loss, stress management, and the sophisticated knowledge of emotional eating become essential aspects of constructing a resilient mindset for long-term success.

The importance of sleep and recovery strategies further enhances our narrative. We reveal the crucial significance of excellent sleep in the weight control equation and give efficient recovery approaches essential for people leading active lifestyles.

As we negotiate the shifting environment, lifestyle adjustments emerge as stalwart companions on this expedition. We study the art of habit development and delve into the crucial role of social support and accountability, acknowledging their transforming power in sustaining positive change.

In this journey, setbacks and plateaus are not just roadblocks but possibilities for progress. We explore tactics for breaking through weight loss plateaus and give thoughts on overcoming setbacks, allowing readers to endure the inevitable peaks and valleys of their own voyage.

This is not a one-size-fits-all recipe but a personalized roadmap for individuals seeking their particular path to transformation. By tailoring techniques to individual requirements and modifying the formula to various lifestyles, we empower readers to travel their own trajectory from fat to fit.

Embedded throughout these book chapters are fascinating case studies—real stories of success, tenacity, and self-discovery. As we go through these anecdotes, we extract essential insights from those who have walked the path, providing actual proof that the shift from fat to fit is not just an aspiration but an achievable reality

So, dear reader, welcome to a discourse that surpasses the commonplace, a narrative fashioned from the strands of knowledge, experience, and steadfast conviction. Embrace this journey with an open mind and a determination to transform, for within this book lies the blueprint to uncover the secrets of comprehensive weight management.

Overview of the Fat to Fit Journey

At the heart of the transformative path from fat to fit is a profound exploration of the various facets of comprehensive weight management. It is a journey not merely characterized by the numbers on a scale but rather, a holistic endeavor incorporating the delicate combination of body, mind, and lifestyle. The process unfolds as an individualized expedition, acknowledging that each person's route to wellness is unique, formed by their specific physiology, experiences, and desires.

It begins with a fundamental grasp of body composition, where the focus expands beyond the standard measures. We navigate the nuances of body fat percentage and muscle mass, realizing that true health transcends simply weight loss and incorporates the cultivation of lean, functional strength. This core information sets the way for a more nuanced and sustainable approach to weight management.

Within the scientific underpinnings of weight loss, we look at the mysteries of metabolism and hormone regulation. This knowledge serves as a compass, guiding us towards informed decisions in nutrition and exercise, therefore helping individuals to manage their journey with clarity and purpose. The discourse is not bound to hard norms but embraces the flexibility required to respond to varied lifestyles and personal preferences.

Nutrition appears as a vital cornerstone in our path. Beyond the usual notion of dieting, we advocate for a balanced and healthful approach. From the selection of nutrient-dense foods to the incorporation of superfoods, the emphasis is on nourishment that fuels the body and promotes long-term health.

Simultaneously, the tale stretches beyond the physical realm, diving into the psychology of weight loss. The importance of mental well-being becomes clear as we untangle the influence of stress, emotional eating, and the building of a resilient attitude. Recognizing that the mind plays a crucial role in shaping habits and sustaining positive change, we address the psychological intricacies that underline the path from fat to fit.

Physical activity, a stalwart partner in this journey, is studied not as a mere responsibility but as a method to develop vitality and build a robust, functional body. The integration of cardiovascular exercises and strength training techniques is offered not as a prescription but as a toolset for individuals to modify according to their interests and goals.

As we go forward, the need for quality sleep and effective recovery measures is highlighted. These factors are not just adjuncts but fundamental components that contribute to the total well-being of an individual, assuring the longevity of the transformative process.

This is not a straight trip with a defined endpoint, but a dynamic progression. Challenges are not hurdling but opportunities for progress, and setbacks become vital chapters in the tale of triumph. With a commitment to recognizing individual triumphs, learning from disappointments, and adapting to changing circumstances, this journey unfolds as a remarkable narrative of self-discovery, perseverance, and enduring transformation.

The Importance of Comprehensive Weight Management

The relevance of comprehensive weight management extends far beyond the goal of a desirable look; it involves a tremendous impact on total health and well-being. At its core, this approach emphasizes that obtaining and maintaining a healthy weight is not a one-dimensional undertaking but a dynamic process that encompasses several interconnected parts of an individual's life.

Health, both physical and mental, is closely tied to body weight. The importance of maintaining a healthy weight range cannot be overemphasized, since it directly influences the risk of chronic diseases such as diabetes, cardiovascular difficulties, and some malignancies. Beyond the immediate health hazards, there is a dramatic ripple effect on one's quality of life, with consequences for mobility, energy levels, and lifespan.

Comprehensive weight management transcends the constraints of short-term remedies or fad diets. It is a sustainable, lifestyle-oriented strategy that addresses the varied nature of an individual's well-being. By recognizing the relationship between nutrition, physical exercise, mental health, and sleep, this method targets the fundamental causes of weight-related difficulties, enabling permanent improvement.

Nutrition, as a key component, plays a pivotal role in this paradigm. It is not just about caloric restriction but also fueling the body with the correct balance of nutrients. A well-rounded, balanced diet offers the foundation for prolonged energy, good physical processes, and the retention of lean muscle mass throughout weight loss.

Physical activity is another cornerstone, providing not just a tool to burn calories but also a catalyst for improved cardiovascular health, enhanced metabolism, and the growth of lean muscle. This method reframes exercise as a pleasurable and important part of daily life, encouraging individuals to discover activities that correspond with their tastes and goals.

Mental well-being, typically disregarded in conventional weight control conversations, is given proper significance. Stress management, emotional well-being, and the formation of a positive mentality are regarded as essential variables that influence lifestyle choices, habits, and overall success in the weight management journey.

Moreover, comprehensive weight management understands the need for regular sleep and appropriate recovery measures. The healing capacity of sleep is not only crucial for overall health but also affects hormone balance and metabolic activities. Incorporating efficient recovery practices ensures that the body is resilient, lowering the danger of burnout and injuries associated with rigorous physical activities.

The relevance of comprehensive weight control lies in its holistic approach. It understands that obtaining and maintaining a healthy weight is not an isolated goal but a reflection of a balanced and happy lifestyle. By addressing the multiple components of well-being in unison, this method helps individuals not just shed extra weight but also create enduring habits that contribute to a healthier, more happy life.

Chapter 1

Understanding Body Composition

Understanding body composition is a vital component of the journey toward holistic health and effective weight management. It goes beyond the typical focus on body weight, bringing light to the delicate balance between many components that compose human bodies. Body composition is simply the breakdown of these components, notably distinguishing between body fat and lean mass, delivering a more accurate depiction of one's physical status than a mere scale reading.

Body fat percentage acts as a crucial statistic in this investigation. It delineates the fraction of total body weight constituted of fat, providing insights into the distribution and health implications of adipose tissue. An optimal body fat percentage is not only vital for aesthetics but is crucial in minimizing the dangers connected with obesity-related health issues.

Conversely, understanding muscle mass is also crucial. Beyond its role in enabling movement and strength, lean muscle mass contributes significantly to metabolic rate. The preservation and development of muscle become key components in weight management, as they play a pivotal role in supporting overall health and vigor.

Recognizing the significance of lean mass above conventional weight measurements, body composition analysis becomes a more accurate judge of progress. Aiming for a balance between fat loss and muscle retention ensures that weight control efforts are not impaired by the depletion of critical lean tissue.

In the quest for healthy body composition, it is crucial to understand that there is no one-size-fits-all method. Factors such as age, gender, genetics, and lifestyle contribute to individual variances. The focus moves from reaching an arbitrary ideal weight to attaining a tailored balance that matches with an individual's unique physiology and health goals.

Practical methods such as bioelectrical impedance analysis (BIA), dual-energy x-ray absorptiometry (DXA), and skinfold calipers provide quantitative insights into body composition. Utilizing these tools, individuals can modify their techniques, assuring a targeted and effective approach to weight management. This comprehensive understanding of body composition helps individuals to make informed decisions regarding nutrition, exercise, and general lifestyle, supporting a sustained and tailored route toward optimal health and well-being.

Body Fat Percentage Demystified

Body fat %, an important parameter in the field of body composition, serves as a key predictor of an individual's general health and fitness. Demystifying this topic includes recognizing that body fat percentage is not only a cosmetic concern but a significant indication of one's well-being. It shows the fraction of total body weight constituted of fat tissue, encompassing both necessary and stored fats.

The relevance of body fat % rests in its position as a more insightful metric than the usual scale reading. While total body weight provides a numerical figure, it fails to distinguish between fat and lean mass, missing the nuanced makeup of the human body. A higher body fat percentage is associated with increased health risks, including cardiovascular difficulties, diabetes, and other obesity-related illnesses.

Achieving an optimal body fat percentage is not a one-size-fits-all approach. Factors such as age, gender, genetics, and lifestyle contribute to individual variances. What may be considered a healthy range for one individual may differ for another. Thus, the goal becomes a personalized approach that corresponds with each individual's unique physiology and health objectives.

Striking a balance between essential fat, which is necessary for regular physiological activities, and stored fat, which can pose health hazards in excess, is a major factor. Essential fat contributes to hormone balance, insulation, and cushioning of organs. However, excessive body fat, particularly in visceral areas, can lead to health concerns.

Practical methods such as bioelectrical impedance analysis (BIA) and skinfold calipers aid in estimating body fat percentage. These technologies offer vital insights into the distribution of fat around the body. While no measurement method is ideal, these instruments provide a valuable standard for tracking changes over time, allowing individuals to refine their tactics for optimal weight management.

Understanding body fat percentage demystifies the search for a healthier physique. It moves the focus from a concern on numbers to a more holistic examination of total well-being. Embracing the notion that maintaining a healthy body composition is a dynamic and individualized process empowers individuals to make informed decisions regarding their nutrition, activity, and lifestyle, creating a sustainable and tailored route toward optimal health.

Muscle Mass and its Role in Weight Management

Muscle mass, typically downplayed in conversations focused on weight management, emerges as a vital component in the intricate landscape of body composition. Beyond its role in aiding movement and power, muscle mass plays a significant part in the dynamics of efficient weight management. It is not only a cosmetic consideration but a functional asset that substantially affects an individual's metabolic rate and overall well-being.

The metabolic element of muscle hypertrophy is particularly notable. Unlike adipose tissue, which is physiologically less active, lean muscle requires more energy for maintenance. As a result, persons with more muscle mass tend to have a higher basal metabolic rate (BMR), meaning they burn more calories at rest. This natural property of muscle gives a significant advantage in weight management attempts, contributing to more effective calorie usage.

Moreover, the preservation and development of muscle become paramount during weight loss initiatives. Traditional treatments focusing primarily on calorie reduction may accidentally lead to the loss of both fat and muscle. However, acknowledging the relevance of muscle in weight management suggests a more nuanced technique. Prioritizing protein consumption and implementing strength training exercises become vital components of a comprehensive strategy, ensuring that the weight lost largely includes fat rather than lean tissue.

The benefits of muscle extend beyond its metabolic prowess. Lean muscle mass serves a key function in supporting joint health, boosting overall mobility, and reinforcing the body against injuries. Additionally, the aesthetic factor, frequently a secondary consideration, becomes an extra drive for individuals pursuing weight management. Well-defined muscles contribute to a toned figure, promoting a sense of accomplishment and enhancing self-confidence.

Practical solutions for improving muscle mass need a complex approach. Resistance training exercises, covering weightlifting and bodyweight workouts, serve to enhance muscle growth. Coupled with a proper diet of protein, necessary amino acids fuel the repair and growth of muscle tissue. This symbiotic interaction between nutrition and exercise constitutes the basis of a balanced strategy for growing and sustaining lean muscle mass.

Muscle mass is not only a passive component of the body but an active contributor to healthy weight management. By appreciating its significance in metabolic function, mobility, and overall health, individuals can customize their approach to weight loss with an emphasis on conserving and increasing lean muscle. This understanding alters the narrative from a sole concentration on shedding pounds to a holistic quest for ideal body composition and well-being.

Chapter 2

The Science Behind Weight Loss

The science behind weight reduction is a dynamic and varied field, going into the physiological processes that determine how our bodies absorb and store energy. At its foundation, weight loss rests on the simple yet profound principle of creating an energy deficit — burning more calories than consumed. This process, however, is far from elementary, comprising a complex interaction of metabolic, hormonal, and behavioral components.

Metabolism, generally described as the body's engine, is a critical player in the weight reduction equation. It encompasses the processes by which the body turns food into energy and expends that energy for numerous physiological tasks. Understanding the complexity of metabolism sheds light on why individuals may have variances in how they respond to food changes and exercise.

Hormones, the messengers that govern numerous body activities, play a crucial role in weight regulation. Insulin, for instance, encourages the storage of carbohydrates as fat, whereas hormones like leptin and ghrelin signal hunger and satiety. A full understanding of these hormonal reactions provides insights into why some individuals may struggle with weight loss despite strenuous efforts, stressing the significance of personalized approaches tailored to individual hormonal profiles.

Beyond the common wisdom of "calories in, calories out," the quality of calories ingested also determines weight reduction outcomes. Not all calories are created equal, and the source of these calories can affect metabolism, appetite, and overall energy balance. The content of a diet, prioritizing nutrient-dense foods over empty-calorie choices, becomes a significant issue in the scientific approach to weight management.

The concept of the "set point," a weight range in which the body naturally maintains, further elucidates the issues individuals encounter in losing and maintaining weight. The body's innate defense mechanisms, meant to conserve energy supplies, can oppose attempts at prolonged weight loss. Acknowledging this biological inclination influences the creation of tactics that go beyond short-term remedies, concentrating on sustainable lifestyle improvements.

Scientifically informed weight loss strategies expand beyond the typical emphasis on diet and exercise. The importance of sleep in weight regulation, for example, is gaining significance. Sleep deprivation can disturb the hormonal balance, leading to increased hunger and poor glucose metabolism, ultimately harming weight management attempts.

The science behind weight loss is a continual inquiry, incorporating knowledge from physiology, diet, and behavioral psychology. It underlines the necessity for tailored methods that account for the individual's metabolic profile, hormone responses, and lifestyle factors. As our grasp of these fundamental concepts grows, so too does our ability to devise more effective and individualized solutions for achieving and maintaining healthy weight goals.

Metabolism and its Impact on Fat Burning

Metabolism, sometimes equated to the body's internal engine, is a complex network of biochemical reactions that transform food into energy to sustain numerous physiological functions. Its impact on fat burning is substantial, functioning as a vital role in the complicated balance of energy expenditure and storage inside the human body.

The basal metabolic rate (BMR) is a key element of metabolism, representing the energy expended at rest to maintain essential body activities such as breathing, circulation, and cell formation. Understanding BMR is vital since it establishes the baseline for the calories burned throughout the day. Individuals with a higher BMR naturally burn more calories, contributing to more efficient fat burning.

The thermic effect of food (TEF), another component of metabolism, represents the energy expended during the digestion and absorption of food. Different macronutrients nessed varying amounts of energy for digestion. Protein, for instance, has a stronger thermic impact compared to fats and carbs, meaning the body expends more energy processing protein-rich diets, perhaps aiding in fat burning.

Physical activity, including both purposeful exercise and daily movements, contributes greatly to metabolism and fat burning. Regular exercise not only burns calories during the activity itself but also has a lasting impact on metabolism by boosting the development and maintenance of lean muscle mass. Muscles, being metabolically active, enhance the body's overall energy expenditure, enhancing the capacity for fat burning.

The significance of hormones in metabolism further highlights its impact on fat burning. Insulin, for example, affects glucose metabolism and fat accumulation. When insulin sensitivity is maximized through factors like regular exercise and a balanced diet, the body is better suited to properly utilize glucose for energy, minimizing the likelihood of excess glucose being deposited as fat.

Moreover, the relationship between metabolism and fat burning is controlled by factors beyond diet and exercise. Adequate sleep plays a vital role in hormone regulation, particularly impacting leptin and ghrelin, which control hunger and satiety. Disrupted sleep habits can disturb these hormonal balances, potentially leading to increased appetite and hampered fat burning.

Metabolism's impact on fat burning is a dynamic and diverse process. While factors like genetics and age contribute to individual variances in metabolic rate, lifestyle choices play a key influence in optimizing metabolism for effective fat burning. A holistic strategy, incorporating nutrition, exercise, and sleep, is crucial to maintaining a metabolic state conducive to sustainable and healthy fat loss.

Hormones and Weight Regulation

Hormones play a key role in the complicated game of weight management within the human body. These chemical messengers compose a symphony of signals that impact hunger, satiety, metabolism, and the storage of fat. Understanding the delicate balance of these hormones is vital for deciphering the complexity of weight management.

Insulin, frequently related to blood sugar regulation, plays a prominent role in the field of weight control. It enhances the absorption of glucose by cells for energy usage or storage. However, when insulin sensitivity is reduced, as typically observed in disorders like insulin resistance, excess glucose can be stored as fat, resulting in weight gain. Maintaining insulin sensitivity through lifestyle factors, including regular exercise and a balanced diet, is crucial in fostering good weight regulation.

Leptin and ghrelin, sometimes referred to as the hunger hormones, play a vital role in appetite control. Leptin, produced by fat cells, signals to the brain that the body has sufficient energy stores, causing a feeling of fullness. On the other hand, ghrelin, produced in the stomach, activates hunger signals. An imbalance in these hormones can contribute to overeating and, subsequently, weight gain. Strategies that enhance hormonal balance, such as appropriate sleep and stress management, contribute to healthier appetite regulation.

Cortisol, the stress hormone, is another member of the hormonal orchestra with consequences for weight management. Elevated cortisol levels, a frequent response to prolonged stress, can contribute to increased hunger, particularly for high-calorie foods. This stress-induced eating, coupled with the body's tendency to retain excess calories as fat during stress, underlines the complicated relationship between emotional well-being and weight management.

Sex hormones, including estrogen and testosterone, also influence weight distribution and metabolism. Hormonal shifts during different life stages, such as menopause or andropause, might alter body composition and the inclination to gain weight, especially around the abdomen area. Recognizing these hormonal swings and adopting lifestyle choices to reduce their impact is vital for maintaining a healthy weight.

Hormones comprise a dynamic regulatory system that intimately regulates weight regulation. The delicate balance of insulin, leptin, ghrelin, cortisol, and sex hormones dictates how the body stores and utilizes energy. Nurturing hormonal health by lifestyle choices, including a balanced diet, regular exercise, appropriate sleep, and stress management, becomes a significant technique in encouraging efficient weight regulation.

Chapter 3

Building a Solid Foundation: Nutrition Essentials

To lay a solid foundation for weight management, it is necessary to place a strong emphasis on aspects of diet that are crucial. It entails building a sustainable and balanced approach that nourishes the body while supporting the quest for health and vitality. This goes beyond the usual conceptions of dieting so that it may be considered a more holistic approach.

The idea of developing a food plan that is well-balanced is essential to the foundation of this foundation. It is vital to maintain a balance of macronutrients, which include proteins, carbs, and fats, in order to fulfill the various nutritional requirements of the body. Proteins, essential for the growth and repair of muscle tissue, can be obtained from lean meats, dairy products, and plant-based alternatives. Fruits, vegetables, and grains that are whole are all good sources of carbohydrates, which are the major source of energy for the body. Avocados, almonds, and olive oil are all examples of foods that contain these healthy fats, which are essential for the generation of hormones and the absorption of nutrients.

The acknowledgment of the significance of micronutrients, which include vitamins and minerals, is also of equal importance. The consumption of a diet that is abundant in colorful fruits and vegetables offers a wide range of vital nutrients, which contributes to an overall sense of well-being. Assuring that the body receives the full spectrum of vitamins and minerals that are essential for optimal functioning can be accomplished by consuming a wide range of foods that are rich in nutrients.

The emphasis on superfoods adds a significant dimension to dietary essentials. These nutrient-packed foods, such as berries, leafy greens, and fatty fish, offer an abundance of antioxidants, omega-3 fatty acids, and other health-promoting substances. Integrating superfoods into the diet delivers a significant boost to general health and aids weight-control goals.

Portion control is a crucial part of nutrition essentials. In a culture generally accustomed to enormous servings, identifying optimal portion sizes is crucial to minimizing the overconsumption of calories. cues Mindful eating and paying attention to hunger and fullness cues, further adds to creating a good connection with food and supports sustained weight management.

Hydration, frequently disregarded in weight management talks, is crucial to nutrition needs. Water plays a key part in metabolism, digestion, and overall body processes. Adequate hydration aids in satiety, reducing the chance of overeating, and promotes the body's natural cleansing processes.

The concept of dietary basics extends beyond restrictive diets or temporary remedies. It entails building a long-term, healthy connection with food, and realizing that each individual's nutritional demands are unique. Customizing nutritional methods based on personal preferences, cultural influences, and health considerations contributes to the durability and success of a nutrition plan.

Building a firm foundation through nutrition essentials is about creating a holistic and balanced approach to food. It is not about deprivation but rather about making informed choices that align with health and well-being. By embracing the concepts of balance, diversity, and moderation, individuals can create the framework for a lasting and healthy relationship with food, crucial for the road toward effective weight management.

Creating a Balanced Diet Plan

Crafting a balanced food plan is a crucial cornerstone in the pursuit of good nutrition and effective weight management. It entails a strategic selection and mix of foods that supply the necessary nutrients for overall health while supporting specific goals like weight loss or muscle building.

At the basis of a balanced meal plan is the consideration of macronutrients - proteins, carbs, and fats. Proteins, important for muscle repair and growth, can be sourced from lean meats, poultry, fish, dairy, and plant-based choices like lentils and tofu. Carbohydrates, the body's major energy source, are found in fruits, vegetables, whole grains, and legumes. Healthy fats, necessary for hormone production and nutrition absorption, are abundant in avocados, nuts, seeds, and olive oil.

The distribution of these macronutrients within the diet is crucial. While individual needs may vary, a balanced diet typically incorporates a reasonable consumption of proteins, a range of colorful fruits and vegetables for carbs, and sources of healthy fats in appropriate amounts. Achieving this balance not only delivers critical nutrients but also aids in building an enjoyable and sustainable eating plan.

Micronutrients, including vitamins and minerals, play a key role in supporting general health. A vast and colorful array of fruits and vegetables enables the absorption of a broad spectrum of these necessary elements. Nutrient-dense foods such as leafy greens, berries, and cruciferous vegetables contribute not only to the body's nutritional needs but also to its resilience against many health concerns.

Superfoods, rich in antioxidants, omega-3 fatty acids, and other health-promoting substances, can be deliberately incorporated into a balanced diet plan. These nutrient powerhouses, ranging from berries and dark leafy greens to fatty fish and nuts, offer extra advantages that boost general well-being.

Portion control is a vital part of creating a balanced diet plan. Understanding optimal portion sizes reduces the overconsumption of calories, contributing to weight management. Mindful eating, characterized by paying attention to hunger and fullness cues, further enhances portion control and fosters a healthier connection with food.

Hydration, frequently overlooked, is a vital aspect of a balanced food plan. Water plays a key part in digestion, metabolism, and overall body processes. Incorporating a proper amount of water into daily routines adds to satiety, reducing the likelihood of overeating.

Creating a balanced diet plan is about more than just calculating calories or following rigorous limits. It comprises embracing a range of nutrient-dense meals, creating a harmonious balance between macronutrients, and acknowledging the necessity of portion control and hydration. By tailoring this diet based on individual preferences and nutritional needs, individuals can establish the foundation for a sustainable and satisfying approach to eating, supporting their path toward optimal health and weight management.

Superfoods for Sustainable Weight Loss

Superfoods, lauded for their nutrient richness and health-promoting capabilities, appear as helpful friends in the fight for sustainable weight loss within the field of dietary fundamentals. These nutritional powerhouses, rich in vitamins, minerals, antioxidants, and other beneficial substances, offer a strategic addition to a well-balanced diet.

Berries, especially blueberries, strawberries, and raspberries, stand out as excellent superfoods. Packed with antioxidants, fiber, and vitamins, these colorful jewels not only assist in general health but also support weight management by giving a pleasant and naturally sweet addition to meals and snacks.

Leafy greens, such as kale, spinach, and Swiss chard, are nutritious powerhouses that merit a prominent role in any diet focused on weight loss. High in fiber, low in calories, and abundant in critical vitamins and minerals, these greens deliver a nutrient boost while generating a feeling of fullness, aiding with calorie control.

Fatty fish, such as salmon, mackerel, and trout, bring omega-3 fatty acids to the table. These good fats not only improve cardiovascular health but also play a role in inducing satiety and lowering inflammation, making them ideal partners in a weight loss journey.

Quinoa, frequently considered a "super grain," is a complete protein source containing all essential amino acids. This gluten-free grain provides continuous energy, making it a perfect choice for individuals seeking a nutrient-dense and enjoyable supplement to their meals.

Nuts and seeds, including almonds, chia seeds, and flaxseeds, are rich in healthy fats, fiber, and protein. Incorporating them into the diet not only provides a crunchy texture but also contributes to a feeling of fullness, lowering the likelihood of overeating.

Avocados, frequently recognized for their creamy texture, offer more than simply taste. Packed in monounsaturated fats, avocados contribute to satiety while providing critical nutrients, making them a flexible and healthful addition to salads, sandwiches, or as a stand-alone snack.

Greek yogurt, a protein-packed dairy choice, is not only a delightful snack but also a valuable superfood. With probiotics that support gut health, it adds to general well-being while delivering a tasty and nutrient-dense alternative to a weight-conscious diet.

Incorporating these superfoods into a balanced eating plan gives both diversity and nutritional benefits. Their mix of important nutrients, antioxidants, and satiating characteristics promotes weight loss attempts by increasing overall health, generating a feeling of fullness, and delivering prolonged energy. While no single food can guarantee weight reduction, strategically adding these nutrient-dense foods can contribute to a sustainable and enjoyable strategy for reducing unwanted pounds.

Chapter 4

Crafting an Effective Exercise Routine

Crafting a good exercise regimen is a crucial component of any holistic approach to dietary fundamentals and weight management. Exercise not only contributes to the burning of calories but also plays a key role in increasing metabolism, improving cardiovascular health, and fostering overall well-being.

The first step in building a successful fitness plan is determining individual preferences and goals. Whether it's aerobic exercises like jogging or cycling, strength training with weights, or more holistic techniques like yoga or Pilates, picking activities that correspond with personal interests boosts the likelihood of consistency and commitment to the practice.

Diversification within the exercise program is crucial. Combining aerobic workouts with strength training and flexibility exercises gives a well-rounded strategy that addresses many aspects of fitness. This complete technique not only assists weight loss but also contributes to general physical health and functional fitness.

Setting realistic and achievable goals is key in keeping motivation and measuring progress. Whether aiming for a set number of weekly sessions, a specific time of exercise, or progressive increases in intensity, having tangible goals delivers a sense of direction and success.

Consistency is crucial in any effective fitness plan. Rather than focusing on rare intensive exercises, establishing a regular program that integrates exercise into daily life supports habit formation. This steady strategy adds to long-term success in weight management and general health.

Considering individual fitness levels and progressively rising in intensity is crucial. Sudden and severe shifts might lead to fatigue or injury. A gradual increase in the duration, intensity, or complexity of exercises helps the body to adapt and minimizes the danger of setbacks.

Cross-training, or incorporating multiple types of exercise, not only minimizes monotony but also prevents overuse problems linked with repetitive actions. Mixing high-intensity workouts with lower-intensity activities boosts recuperation and preserves long-term involvement.

Recognizing the symbiotic relationship between exercise and nutrition is fundamental. A well-balanced diet, rich in nutrients, promotes energy levels and recovery, improving the benefits received from the exercise regimen. Adequate hydration is similarly crucial, contributing to good performance and recuperation.

Lastly, getting professional advice, such as working with a certified fitness trainer or consulting a healthcare professional, ensures that the exercise regimen corresponds with individual demands and health considerations. Professional assistance assists in adapting the regimen to personal goals while treating any underlying health concerns.

In a nutshell, building a good fitness regimen needs a thoughtful and tailored approach. By embracing a range of activities, setting realistic objectives, stressing consistency, and recognizing the synergy between exercise and diet, individuals can develop sustainable habits that help not only weight control but also to total physical and emotional well-being.

Cardiovascular Workouts for Fat Burning

Cardiovascular workouts, generally referred to as cardio exercises, play a crucial function in fat burning within the framework of nutrition needs. These workouts, characterized by persistent periods of high heart rate and increased oxygen consumption, help burn calories, enhance cardiovascular health, and help overall weight management.

Engaging in activities such as running, cycling, swimming, or brisk walking boosts the heart rate, commencing a process where the body taps into stored fat as an energy source. This fat-burning component of cardiovascular workouts makes them particularly advantageous for anyone aiming to remove excess pounds or maintain a healthy weight.

The intensity and length of cardiovascular workouts are crucial elements impacting their efficiency in fat burning. While moderate-intensity exercises are sustainable over longer periods, high-intensity interval training (HIIT) has gained appeal for its ability to optimize calorie burn in shorter intervals. HIIT alternates between short bursts of strong work and brief periods of rest or lower intensity, pushing the body and encouraging fat oxidation.

Consistency in cardiovascular activities is key for ongoing fat-burning advantages. Incorporating these workouts into a weekly regimen, whether through dedicated sessions or integrating them into daily activities, contributes to the cumulative calorie deficit necessary for weight loss.

Cardiovascular workouts also extend beyond the acute calorie burn. Regular engagement in these exercises boosts cardiovascular fitness, improves endurance, and contributes to a healthier heart. This holistic approach not only benefits weight management but also improves general well-being.

Combining cardiovascular activities with a healthy diet boosts the fat-burning impact. While exercise helps with calorie expenditure, a nutrient-dense diet offers the essential fuel for optimal performance and supports recovery, boosting the advantages obtained from cardio workouts.

Variety within cardiovascular training reduces monotony and keeps the body engaged. Mixing diverse exercises or varying the intensity and duration helps avoid plateaus and supports continual fat burning. Enjoyable activities boost adherence, converting fitness into a sustainable lifestyle choice.

Before commencing any cardiovascular workout plan, individuals should assess their fitness levels, and any underlying health concerns, and gradually proceed to higher intensities. Consulting with healthcare specialists or fitness experts ensures that the chosen cardio routines coincide with individual needs and goals.

Incorporating aerobic workouts within a well-rounded approach to nutrition needs contributes greatly to fat-burning and weight management. Whether through standard aerobic exercises or novel HIIT sessions, these activities serve as vital instruments in the pursuit of a better body and lifestyle.

Strength Training and Lean Muscle Development

Strength training is an integral part of nutrition fundamentals. assumes a key role in the goal of lean muscle development and effective weight management. Unlike traditional conceptions that equate exercise exclusively with calorie expenditure, strength training goes further, contributing to the preservation and growth of lean muscle mass.

Engaging in strength training entails resistance activities, such as weightlifting, bodyweight exercises, or resistance band workouts, that stress the muscles. The stimulus produced by resistance drives the body to adapt, leading to the development and maintenance of lean muscular tissue. This is particularly significant in weight loss initiatives, as it helps avoid the loss of muscle commonly linked with calorie-restricted diets.

Lean muscle mass is metabolically active, meaning it requires energy for upkeep. This metabolic advantage contributes to an enhanced basal metabolic rate (BMR), allowing individuals with more muscle mass to burn more calories at rest. In the context of weight management, this becomes a great tool, promoting more effective calorie consumption and boosting the overall fat-burning capability.

Nutrition has a crucial role in promoting strength training and lean muscle development. A diet rich in protein is vital, as protein provides the building blocks (amino acids) necessary for muscle repair and growth. Incorporating protein sources such as lean meats, poultry, fish, eggs, dairy, and plant-based choices guarantees an adequate supply of critical amino acids for healthy muscular performance.

The timing of nutrient intake is another concern in the context of strength training. Consuming protein-rich meals or snacks around the time of a strength training session improves muscle protein synthesis and enhances recovery. This strategy ensures that the body gets the necessary nutrients available when the need for muscle repair and growth is at its height.

Consistency in strength training regimens is key for sustained outcomes. Progressive overload, gradually increasing the resistance or intensity of exercises, challenges the muscles and encourages constant adaptability. This not only encourages muscular development but also prevents plateaus in performance.

Balancing strength training with cardiovascular workouts provides a well-rounded approach to health. While strength training focuses on creating lean muscle, cardiovascular routines contribute to overall calorie expenditure and cardiovascular health. The combination of these two techniques ensures a comprehensive strategy for optimal weight management.

Strength training is a dynamic and crucial component of nutrition fundamentals for individuals seeking lean muscle development and weight management. Its impact extends beyond physical appearance, influencing metabolic health and overall well-being. With adequate nutrition, incremental resistance, and a consistent approach, strength training becomes a formidable tool for the goal of a healthier, stronger, and more robust body.

Chapter 5

Mental Wellness in the Fat to Fit Journey

Within the overall structure of the fundamentals of nutrition, mental health plays a pivotal role in the path from fat to fit. In spite of the fact that the emphasis is frequently placed on weight loss and physical activity, the psychological aspects of this journey toward transformation are equally important. Positivity and resiliency are two of the most important factors that contribute considerably to successful weight control and changes in lifestyle that are long-lasting.

To achieve mental well-being during the Fat to Fit journey, it is essential to comprehend and reframe one's perception of food. Fostering a healthy connection with food requires acknowledging its function as a source of nourishment for both the body and the mind. This is in contrast to the traditional view of food as only a source of calories. This adjustment in viewpoint helps to build a healthier attitude toward eating, which in turn encourages mindful decisions and reduces the risk of emotional eating.

When it comes to preserving mental wellness throughout the journey, one of the most important factors is setting goals that are both reasonable and attainable. A sense of satisfaction and motivation can be gained from achieving attainable goals, yet having unrealistic expectations can lead to frustration and failed attempts. To reinforce a good mindset and encourage continued growth, it is beneficial to celebrate even the smallest of wins, whether they are related to nutritional decisions or activity goals.

Self-compassion is a crucial component of mental health, and it should be cultivated actively. Acknowledging that the journey may contain occasional deviations from the plan encourages individuals to overcome setbacks without self-judgment. Embracing a compassionate attitude towards oneself promotes resilience and assists in overcoming hurdles, resulting in a more positive and sustainable approach to the Fat to Fit path.

Mindful eating, characterized by being completely present and engaged with the eating experience, corresponds with mental wellness ideals. This practice develops a deeper connection with food, helping consumers to savor and appreciate each bite. By paying attention to hunger and fullness cues, mindful eating enhances both physical and emotional well-being.

Incorporating stress-management techniques is vital in treating the psychological aspects of the Fat to Fit journey. Stress can alter eating patterns and hamper weight-management efforts. Techniques such as meditation, deep breathing, or engaging in enjoyable hobbies help decrease stress, promote mental resilience, and boost general well-being.

Building a support system contributes greatly to mental wellness during the Fat to Fit journey. Whether through friends, family, or professional assistance, having a network of others who understand and encourage the pursuit of a healthy lifestyle provides emotional support and promotes excellent habits.

Lastly, acknowledging the complex nature of the path and embracing the concept of balance is crucial to mental wellness. Rather than adopting an all-or-nothing mentality, realizing that occasional indulgences or deviations are part of a balanced approach relieves the burden of perfectionism. This understanding fosters a sustained and realistic mindset throughout the transformation process.

Mental wellness is an essential aspect of the Fat to Fit path. By creating a positive mindset, setting reasonable objectives, practicing self-compassion, and implementing stress-management skills, individuals can negotiate the obstacles of weight management with resilience and a holistic approach to well-being.

The Psychology of Weight Loss

Understanding the psychology of weight reduction is crucial in navigating the numerous processes that influence our relationship with food and body image. The mental and emotional sides of the journey from fat to fit are equally significant as the physical components, making it imperative to understand the psychological facets of nutrition fundamentals.

One key part of the psychology of weight loss entails addressing the underlying motivations driving the desire for weight management. While external causes like as social standards and peer pressure may influence, identifying intrinsic incentives, such as improved health, more energy, or enhanced self-esteem, can dramatically impact the sustainability of lifestyle changes.

The importance of habits and behavioral patterns in weight loss cannot be emphasized. Our connection with food is typically affected by deeply ingrained patterns, both conscious and subconscious. Identifying these tendencies and creating new, healthier habits demands a level of self-awareness and a willingness to challenge and alter old behaviors.

The impact of emotions on eating behaviors is an important element of the psychology of weight loss. Emotional eating, whether in response to stress, boredom, or other emotional states, can impede weight management efforts. Developing emotional intelligence and other coping skills is crucial in resolving these tendencies and creating a healthier relationship with food.

Setting realistic and achievable goals is a psychological strategy that adds to sustained motivation and positive outcomes. Unrealistic expectations often lead to frustration and may impede progress. Breaking down major goals into smaller, attainable tasks develops a sense of accomplishment and builds confidence in the ability to achieve long-term success.

The function of self-image and body positivity is crucial in the psychology of weight loss. Cultivating a good and welcoming attitude towards one's body, regardless of its current state, fosters a healthier mental outlook. Focusing on self-care, self-love, and body appreciation promotes an attitude that supports permanent changes and minimizes the risk of engaging in harmful or extreme behaviors.

Social support is a psychological component that substantially influences weight loss initiatives. The importance of friends, family, or a supporting community cannot be underestimated. Sharing goals, struggles, and triumphs with others promotes accountability, encouragement, and a sense of connection, strengthening the psychological resilience required for the trip.

Moreover, the psychology of weight loss highlights the role of attention in eating practices. Paying attention to the sensory experience of eating, identifying hunger and fullness cues, and practicing thankfulness for the sustenance supplied by food creates a thoughtful and intentional attitude to eating, contributing to the overall success of weight management efforts.

The psychology of weight loss is a complex investigation of the mental and emotional factors that influence our actions and attitudes toward nutrition and body image. By delving into intrinsic motivations, reshaping habits, addressing emotional patterns, setting realistic goals, fostering a positive self-image, seeking social support, and practicing mindfulness, individuals can create a psychological foundation that supports sustainable and positive changes in their weight management journey.

Stress Management and Emotional Eating

Understanding the psychology of weight loss is important in navigating the complexity of the fat-to-fit journey within the area of nutrition fundamentals. The human mind plays a crucial part in developing behaviors, attitudes, and habits relating to diet, exercise, and overall health. Unraveling the psychological components of weight loss includes recognizing and addressing many factors that influence decision-making and long-term commitment to healthy practices.

One key part of the psychology of weight loss is the influence of habits and routines on behavior. Habits, whether linked to food choices, meal timings, or exercise regimens, are firmly engrained in daily life. Recognizing and altering these patterns is key for permanent change. Small, consistent improvements over time can lead to the creation of better behaviors that support weight management goals.

The concept of self-efficacy, coined by psychologist Albert Bandura, is another crucial factor in the psychology of weight loss. It refers to an individual's belief in their ability to attain specified goals. Cultivating a sense of self-efficacy entails setting reasonable and achievable goals, celebrating victories, and increasing confidence via gradual progress. A strong feeling of self-efficacy promotes motivation and resilience in the face of obstacles.

The role of motivation in weight loss cannot be emphasized. Motivation, however, is not a constant force but fluctuates throughout time. Understanding the numerous types of motivation, including intrinsic (internal) and extrinsic (external) motivation, helps individuals customize their approach. Focusing on intrinsic motivation, anchored in personal values and happiness, develops a more persistent commitment to healthy activities.

Social support appears as a key impact on the psychology of weight loss. The importance of family, friends, or community in lifestyle choices cannot be ignored. Building a supporting network, whether for accountability, encouragement, or shared activities, maintains the commitment to weight management goals. Social relationships create a sense of belonging and understanding, vital for handling problems.

mentality, notably having a growth mentality, is crucial to the psychology of weight loss. A growth mindset views issues as opportunities for learning and growth rather than insurmountable hurdles. Embracing this mindset encourages perseverance in the face of setbacks, develops a positive attitude toward change, and builds a readiness to adjust techniques for long-term success.

Emotional eating, classically linked to psychological reasons, is a key consideration in weight management. Understanding the triggers behind emotional eating, such as stress, boredom, or melancholy, allows individuals to build healthy coping mechanisms. They are cultivating emotional awareness and discovering other ways to address emotional aids to stop the cycle of emotional eating.

One of the main psychological components in the process of weight loss is the impact of self-perception and body image. How individuals view their bodies can dramatically influence their habits and decisions relating to eating and exercise. Nurturing a positive body image requires understanding and respecting the body's assets and possibilities, irrespective of its current size or shape. Shifting the focus from exterior appearance to overall health and well-being creates a more balanced and sustainable approach to weight management.

The concept of cognitive restructuring plays a vital role in modifying thought processes connected to weight loss.

Often, negative or self-defeating beliefs might inhibit progress. Cognitive restructuring entails identifying and confronting these thoughts, and replacing them with more positive and helpful ones. This technique contributes to building a healthier mindset, lowering emotions of guilt or irritation, and fostering a more flexible approach to weight management.

Building resilience is a psychological ability that is beneficial in the face of failures or hurdles during the weight loss journey. Resilience involves bouncing back from challenges, adapting to change, and feeling purpose and direction. Developing resilience enables individuals to negotiate the inevitable ups and downs, learn from events, and stay dedicated to their long-term goals.

The psychological influence of stress on weight management is significant. Chronic stress can lead to emotional eating, hormone imbalances, and disturbances in sleep habits, all of which can contribute to weight gain. Implementing stress-management practices, such as mindfulness, relaxation exercises, or engaging in joyful activities, can lessen the impact of stress on both mental well-being and physical health.

Mindful decision-making is a cognitive talent that permits individuals to make informed decisions about their nutrition and lifestyle. Mindfulness entails being present in the moment and paying attention to thoughts and feelings without judgment. Applying mindfulness to eating habits, exercise routines, and general lifestyle choices creates a deeper awareness of one's actions, leading to more intentional and health-promoting behaviors.

Finally, recognizing the cyclical nature of behavior change and the potential for relapses is key in the psychology of weight reduction. Understanding that occasional failures do not determine overall development allows individuals to learn from experiences, change their plans, and continue moving forward. Embracing a non-judgmental attitude towards oneself helps persistence and resilience in the quest for health and fitness.

The psychology of weight reduction involves a varied spectrum of cognitive and emotional elements that impact behaviors, habits, and attitudes. By addressing these psychological components alongside nutritional concerns, individuals can construct a comprehensive and sustainable strategy for their fat-to-fit journey. A holistic awareness of the connection between the mind and body helps individuals to make lasting changes that contribute to enhanced overall health and well-being.

Chapter 6

Sleep and Recovery Strategies

Sleep and recovery strategies are essential factors in the pursuit of good health and effective weight management. The importance of adequate sleep cannot be emphasized, as it has a key role in several physiological functions, including hormone balance, metabolism, and overall well-being. Implementing healthy sleep practices is crucial to supporting the body's recovery mechanisms and promoting sustainable development in the fat-to-fit path.

Consistent sleep patterns contribute greatly to overall health. Establishing a regular sleep routine, when one goes to bed and gets up at the same time each day, helps regulate the body's internal clock. This constancy promotes the quality of sleep, allowing individuals to benefit from the complete range of restorative processes that occur during the distinct sleep cycles.

Creating a suitable sleep environment is crucial for optimizing sleep quality. This involves minimizing light exposure, particularly from electronic devices, in the hours preceding bedtime. The body's natural production of melatonin, a sleep-inducing hormone, is regulated by exposure to light. Dimming lights and creating a tranquil, comfortable sleep place contribute to a more restful and restorative night's sleep.

Mindful attention to dietary choices can also affect sleep. Consuming large or heavy meals close to bedtime may interrupt sleep owing to digestive processes. Conversely, including sleep-supportive foods, such as those rich in tryptophan (found in turkey, dairy, and nuts) and magnesium (found in leafy greens, nuts, and seeds), can encourage relaxation and aid in more restful sleep.

Engaging in relaxation exercises before bedtime can boost sleep quality. Practices such as deep breathing, gradual muscular relaxation, or moderate stretching can help reduce tension and communicate to the body that it's time to wind down. Creating a soothing nighttime routine assists in a smoother transition into restful sleep.

Strategies to enhance recovery extend beyond sleep and include focused actions to regenerate the body after physical exertion. Incorporating rest days into a workout plan allows muscles and joints to recuperate, lowering the chance of overuse problems. Active recuperation, incorporating low-intensity activities like walking or moderate yoga, increases circulation and aids in muscle healing.

Hydration is a critical part of both sleep and recovery. Staying appropriately hydrated maintains general health, aids in cellular function, and enables the body's natural recovery processes. Maintaining a steady and balanced intake of fluids throughout the day contributes to healthy hydration levels, thereby improving sleep quality and recovery.

Sleep and recovery strategies represent vital components of a holistic approach to health and weight management. Prioritizing consistent sleep habits, creating a suitable sleep environment, making mindful nutritional choices, engaging in relaxation techniques, incorporating rest days, and being hydrated collectively contribute to an environment that encourages physical and mental well-being. Implementing these measures not only promotes the body's recovery mechanisms but also enhances overall resilience and capacity to overcome the hurdles of the fat-to-fit path.

Importance of Quality Sleep in Weight Management

The importance of adequate sleep in weight management is a component often neglected yet bears deep consequences for general health and well-being. Sleep is not only a passive condition; it is a dynamic process during which the body undertakes necessary repairs, hormone regulation, and cognitive consolidation. When studying the complicated balance of factors influencing weight, the function of adequate, restorative sleep emerges as a vital component.

One of the key processes through which sleep affects weight management is hormone modulation. Sleep deprivation affects the delicate balance of hormones that govern appetite and satiety. Ghrelin, the hormone that drives appetite, increases with poor sleep, while leptin, responsible for signaling fullness, declines. This hormonal imbalance can lead to heightened desires, increased caloric consumption, and an inclination to pick high-calorie, sweet meals.

Beyond hormones, the link between sleep and metabolism is notable. Sleep deficit impacts the body's capacity to control glucose and insulin, potentially leading to insulin resistance and an increased risk of developing type 2 diabetes.

Additionally, poor sleep impairs the metabolism of carbohydrates, contributing to raised blood sugar levels and the accumulation of surplus energy as fat.

The impact of sleep on decision-making and impulse control also plays a role in weight management. Sleep-deprived adults generally demonstrate impaired cognitive function, making it tougher to resist bad eating choices and stick to dietary goals. The combination of heightened desires, impaired decision-making, and a decreased capacity to engage in physical activity can create a cycle that undermines weight management efforts.

Furthermore, the connection between sleep and physical activity is bidirectional. Regular exercise promotes better sleep quality, while the opposite is also true—adequate sleep boosts the capacity for physical activity. Sleep deprivation can lead to weariness and decreased motivation to engage in exercise, affecting the overall energy expenditure needed for weight maintenance.

The psychological implications of sleep cannot be disregarded in the context of weight management. Lack of sleep often results in higher stress levels and emotional sensitivity, resulting in emotional eating and the consumption of comfort foods. Managing stress becomes more problematic with poor sleep, further worsening the influence on dietary choices and general weight-related behaviors.

In a nutshell, acknowledging the symbiotic relationship between sound sleep and weight management is crucial for anyone embarking on a road toward greater health. Prioritizing consistent sleep patterns, providing a sleep-conducive environment, and understanding the multidimensional impact of sleep on hormones, metabolism, decision-making, and emotional well-being collectively contribute to a complete strategy for obtaining and maintaining a healthy weight. The importance of regular sleep in the complicated tapestry of weight management highlights the necessity for a comprehensive strategy that examines both food and lifestyle factors.

Effective Recovery Techniques for Active Lifestyles

Effective recuperation procedures are crucial for those leading active lifestyles, which means they play a pivotal role in maximizing performance, reducing accidents, and supporting long-term well-being. Engaging in regular physical exercise places stress on the body, making the implementation of efficient recovery measures vital for sustaining peak performance and general health.

One key part of optimal rehabilitation is rest days. Incorporating regular rest days into an active program allows the body to repair and replenish. During moments of rest, muscles recover from micro-tears induced by exercise, minimizing the likelihood of overuse problems. A well-balanced exercise schedule, which includes variations in intensity and types of exercises, allows specific muscle areas to rest while others are engaged, improving overall recovery.

Active recovery represents a dynamic approach to recuperation. Light-intensity activities, such as walking, swimming, or moderate yoga, enhance blood circulation and assist in clearing out metabolic wastes, improving the recuperation process. Active recuperation exercises promote flexibility, reduce muscle stiffness, and add to an overall sense of well-being without exerting excessive load on the body.

Incorporating flexibility and mobility exercises into a daily program is another excellent rehabilitation approach. Stretching not only increases flexibility but also helps release muscle tension and lessen the risk of injury. Dynamic stretching before exercise and static stretching post-exercise lead to a greater range of motion, allowing the body to move more efficiently during physical activity.

Nutrition plays a crucial part in optimal rehabilitation. Consuming a well-balanced diet that includes an adequate amount of protein is crucial for muscle repair and growth. Post-exercise diet, particularly during the first hour after a workout, helps replace glycogen levels and aids in the regeneration of injured tissues. Hydration is similarly vital, as it supports multiple physiological activities, including nutrient delivery and temperature regulation.

Cold and heat therapy are well-regarded as excellent rehabilitation techniques. Cold treatments, such as ice baths or cryotherapy, assist in reducing inflammation and alleviate muscle discomfort by restricting blood vessels. Heat therapies, including hot baths or saunas, improve blood flow, relax muscles, and enhance overall recuperation. Alternating between cold and heat techniques, known as contrast therapy, can offer full benefits.

Quality sleep stands as a cornerstone in effective recuperation for active adults. During sleep, the body releases growth hormone, a critical element in muscle repair and recovery. Adequate sleep duration and quality contribute to the restoration of energy levels, better immunological function, and overall mental well-being. Creating a suitable sleep environment and prioritizing consistent sleep patterns are crucial components of a solid recovery approach.

Finally, stress management strategies, such as meditation, deep breathing exercises, or mindfulness practices, are valuable tools in effective rehabilitation. Chronic stress can hamper the body's ability to recuperate by rising cortisol levels, disrupting sleep, and adding to overall weariness. Integrating stress-reducing exercises into a routine boosts the body's resilience and promotes the recovery process.

The use of good healing procedures is crucial to continuing an active lifestyle. By incorporating rest days, embracing active recovery, prioritizing flexibility exercises, maintaining a balanced diet, utilizing cold and heat therapies, prioritizing quality sleep, and implementing stress management techniques, individuals can optimize their recovery, minimize the risk of injuries, and cultivate long-term well-being in the pursuit of an active and healthy lifestyle.

Chapter 7

Lifestyle Changes for Long-Term Success

Implementing lifestyle modifications is a cornerstone for achieving long-term success in any health and wellness quest. While short-term remedies may offer temporary improvements, genuine transformation requires a sustained and holistic approach that incorporates numerous elements of everyday life.

Dietary adjustments stand out as a vital ingredient in sustaining long-term success. Rather than succumbing to restricted diets, adopting a balanced and nutrient-dense eating pattern is vital. Incorporating a range of whole meals, including fruits, vegetables, lean meats, and whole grains, delivers important nutrients and enhances general well-being. Making modest improvements to eating patterns, such as decreasing processed foods and controlling portion sizes, creates a more sustainable approach to nutrition.

Regular physical activity is vital to maintaining a healthy lifestyle over the long term. Instead of perceiving exercise as a transitory chore, integrating enjoyable activities into everyday routines builds a consistent habit. Finding kinds of exercise that correspond with personal interests, whether it's walking, dancing, or engaging in sports, promotes adherence and makes physical activity a joyful part of life.

Cultivating mindfulness in everyday behaviors contributes greatly to long-term success. Mindful eating, which involves paying attention to hunger and fullness signs and savoring each meal, creates a healthier connection with food. Additionally, mindfulness in other aspects of life, such as managing stress or making conscious decisions, helps the general well-being necessary for sustained achievement.

Creating a supportive environment is a critical part of long-term success. Surrounding oneself with positive influences, whether it is friends, family, or a community of like-minded folks, develops encouragement and accountability. Sharing objectives and progress with others provides a network of support that can be essential in overcoming hurdles and celebrating triumphs.

Prioritizing sleep is commonly underestimated in its impact on long-term health. Establishing stable sleep patterns and having a suitable sleep environment contribute to general well-being. Quality sleep improves physical and mental healing, enhances cognitive function, and plays a critical role in sustaining energy levels for sustained success in daily activities.

Stress management is another key component of a lifestyle aimed towards long-term success. Chronic stress can impede health goals by influencing behaviors such as emotional eating or altering sleep patterns. Incorporating stress-reducing activities, such as meditation, deep breathing exercises, or indulging in hobbies, fosters a balanced and resilient approach to daily obstacles.

Embracing a growth mentality is crucial for long-term success. Viewing setbacks as opportunities for learning and growth rather than insurmountable obstacles builds resilience and adaptation. Celebrating minor successes along the way and appreciating progress, no matter how tiny encourages a positive and motivated view of the journey.

long-term success in health and wellness is rooted in the cultivation of sustainable habits throughout all parts of life. By adopting a balanced and nutrient-dense diet, integrating regular physical activity, practicing mindfulness, creating a supportive environment, prioritizing sleep, managing stress effectively, and embracing a growth mindset, individuals can lay the foundation for lasting transformation and a fulfilling and healthy lifestyle.

Habit Formation and Sustainable Weight Maintenance

Habit building is a keystone in the route towards sustainable weight maintenance. Developing healthy habits requires cultivating behaviors that become embedded in daily routines, creating a basis for long-term success. Instead than depending on short-lived improvements, cultivating behaviors that match with overall health goals is vital for permanent weight management.

Initiating habit development frequently begins with setting clear and reasonable goals. Establishing specified, measurable, attainable, relevant, and time-bound (SMART) objectives provides a blueprint for behavioral adjustments. Breaking down larger goals into smaller, attainable steps boosts the feasibility of implementing new habits into daily life.

Consistency is a feature of good habit building. Repeating acts often serves to reinforce brain pathways, making the actions more natural over time. Whether it's choosing healthier dietary choices, engaging in regular exercise, or prioritizing proper sleep, consistency is crucial to ingraining these behaviors into the fabric of one's daily.

Implementing positive reinforcement tactics is crucial in cementing new habits. Celebrating minor successes and praising progress, no matter how tiny, fosters the sensation of accomplishment. This positive feedback loop encourages individuals to continue repeating the desired actions, producing a reinforcing cycle for persistent habit formation.

Habit formation thrives on cue and reward systems. Identifying triggers that activate the desired action and linking them with positive rewards increases the habit loop. For example, if the cue is feeling pressured, engaging in a stress-relief activity like deep breathing or taking a brief walk might serve as a gratifying response, reinforcing the habit of stress management without turning to maladaptive coping techniques.

Creating a supportive atmosphere is a catalyst for good habit formation. Surrounding oneself with cues that inspire positive behaviors and removing impediments that prevent them accelerates the process. This can mean organizing the kitchen for healthy food, scheduling workout sessions in advance, or setting a bedtime routine conducive to great sleep.

Habit formation is an evolutionary process that involves patience and adaptability. Recognizing that setbacks are a natural part of the journey allows individuals to learn from experiences and change methods accordingly. Adopting a growth mindset, which views problems as opportunities for learning and improvement, builds resilience and fortifies the commitment to sustainable habits.

The art of habit building is a dynamic and strategic approach to reaching and maintaining weight management goals. By setting SMART objectives, cultivating consistency, adding positive reinforcement, leveraging cue and reward systems, creating a supportive environment, and embracing a growth mindset, individuals can develop enduring habits that lead to sustainable weight maintenance and general well-being.

Social Support and Accountability

Social support and accountability are linchpins in the fabric of successful health and wellness activities, especially in the context of weight management. Establishing a comprehensive support system can dramatically improve an individual's capacity to achieve sustained lifestyle adjustments. It goes beyond personal willpower and taps into the power of shared goals, support, and community accountability.

At its foundation, social support means soliciting the assistance and encouragement of friends, family, or like-minded persons on the journey towards health. Sharing objectives and progress with a supporting network promotes a sense of camaraderie and understanding. This shared experience gives a significant emotional anchor throughout both victories and challenges.

Accountability, in tandem with social support, provides a dimension of dedication and responsibility to one's health journey. Knowing that others are engaged in one's achievement produces a sense of obligation, driving individuals to adhere to their goals. This shared commitment generates a sort of accountability that extends beyond personal motives, improving the chance of adherence to better practices.

Group dynamics have a vital role in social support and accountability. Engaging in activities such as group exercises, wellness challenges, or regular check-ins creates a shared experience that supports the pursuit of health goals. The combined energy of a supportive group can be a powerful motivator, producing a positive feedback loop that supports regular efforts toward weight management.

The emotional support supplied by a social network is equally crucial. Weight control typically requires managing hurdles, failures, and times of self-doubt. Having individuals who understand the journey and offer empathy, support, and practical counsel can be a cornerstone for resilience and mental well-being.

Technology has also become a key tool in building social support and accountability. Virtual communities, fitness applications, and online forums link folks with shared aspirations, regardless of physical proximity. This digital support system provides a venue for sharing experiences, asking for assistance, and celebrating triumphs, maintaining a sense of community and accountability.

In the workplace, building a culture of health and wellness further enhances the impact of social support and accountability. Implementing wellness programs, organizing group activities, or developing wellness challenges within the workplace creates a collaborative commitment to health. The employment environment becomes a source of encouragement, reinforcing beneficial practices that lead to weight management.

Ultimately, the integration of social support and accountability transforms the quest for health into a shared activity. By enlisting the encouragement of a supporting network, embracing group dynamics, harnessing technology, and building a workplace culture of wellness, individuals can boost their capacity to traverse the challenges of weight control. Social support and accountability become not merely components of a health journey but important threads in the fabric of a supportive and collaborative approach to long-term well-being.

Chapter 8

Overcoming Plateaus and Challenges

Overcoming plateaus and hurdles is an inherent part of any health and wellness journey, particularly in the goal of weight management. Plateaus might be depressing, but they are not insurmountable challenges. Understanding the factors contributing to plateaus and having effective techniques to navigate them is vital for continuous success.

Plateaus often emerge due to the body's tolerance to changes in food and exercise. Initially, significant weight reduction or fitness gains may occur, but over time, the body adjusts, and progress may stall. This is a natural physiological response, and acknowledging it as such is the first step in overcoming plateaus. Patience and a realistic approach become crucial during these stages.

Diversifying both food and exercise regimens is a vital tactic in overcoming plateaus. Introducing variation stops the body from growing too acclimated to precise patterns, potentially jumpstarting improvement. In terms of diet, researching new healthy foods or modifying macronutrient ratios can be advantageous. Similarly, changing the intensity, length, or type of exercise challenges the body in unique ways.

Regularly reassessing goals is another good technique. As individuals achieve progress, their initial goals may alter or require adjustment. Setting new, achievable objectives provides renewed enthusiasm and a clear route forward. This adaptive goal-setting strategy guarantees that individuals remain engaged and dedicated to their health journey.

Addressing the psychological components of plateaus is as crucial. Frustration and discouragement are frequent feelings during these times, and it's vital to establish a resilient mindset. Shifting the attention from the scale to non-scale successes, like as higher energy levels, greater mood, or increased strength, emphasizes the good aspects of the trip.

Seeking professional help, whether from a nutritionist, personal trainer, or mental health professional, can be instrumental in overcoming plateaus. These specialists may provide specific advice, highlight areas that may need change, and offer help targeted to particular needs. Their knowledge gives a significant layer of help during hard moments.

In addition to plateaus, unforeseen challenges may develop, such as lifestyle upheavals, stress, or unexpected setbacks.

Navigating these issues demands agility and a proactive approach. Having contingency preparations, prioritizing self-care during stressful situations, and reframing setbacks as learning opportunities help to resilience in the face of adversities.

Consistency is a cornerstone throughout the journey. Maintaining good practices during plateaus and challenges, even if progress appears stuck, encourages a great lifestyle. Small, regular efforts compound over time, establishing the foundation for long-term success. Embracing the journey as a continuous process, with its ebbs and flows, creates a sustainable and resilient attitude to health and wellness.

Overcoming plateaus and hurdles is a vital element of the dynamic process of weight management. By identifying the factors contributing to plateaus, diversifying routines, reassessing goals, establishing a resilient mindset, obtaining professional help, and maintaining consistency, individuals can navigate through these phases and continue working towards their health objectives.

Identifying and Breaking Through Weight Loss Plateaus

Identifying and breaking through weight loss plateaus is a common problem experienced by individuals attempting to attain their fitness objectives. A plateau occurs when progress seems to stagnate, and the scale remains static despite continued attempts. Recognizing the indicators of a plateau is the first step in resolving this challenge.

One of the symptoms of a weight reduction plateau is a lengthy time of stagnant scale readings. After initial progress, individuals may discover that their weight levels are off, even while they continue with their diet and exercise regimens. While occasional fluctuations are typical, a constant lack of change may signify a plateau.

Plateaus can be ascribed to the body's adaptability to changes in food and exercise. When the body becomes accustomed to a specific habit, it may modify its metabolism and energy expenditure. This adaptive reaction can lead to a slowdown in the rate of weight loss. Understanding that plateaus are a natural part of the weight loss journey is vital for having a positive outlook.

Diversifying both food and exercise routines is a vital approach to breaking past plateaus. Introducing diversity prevents the body from settling into a pattern and boosts its receptivity to change. In terms of food, adjusting calorie intake, experimenting with nutrient distribution, or adopting intermittent fasting can provide a metabolic boost. Likewise, increasing the intensity, length, or style of exercise can encourage the body to overcome stagnation.

Regularly tracking and reassessing food patterns is vital during a plateau. Individuals may accidentally fall into patterns of consuming excess calories or disregarding key components of their nutrition. Keeping a food journal or using tracking apps can shed light on dietary patterns, making it easier to discover areas for modification. Fine-tuning the mix of macronutrients and changing meal sizes may be necessary to rekindle progress.

Implementing high-intensity interval training (HIIT) or integrating strength training routines can be useful in breaking past plateaus. These forms of exercise increase the metabolism and promote fat reduction while keeping lean muscular mass. The use of resistance exercise not only contributes to weight loss but also increases overall body composition.

Addressing stress levels is another key part of overcoming plateaus. Chronic stress can boost cortisol levels, altering hormonal balance and thus impeding weight reduction. Incorporating stress-reducing practices such as mindfulness, meditation, or yoga can contribute to breaking through plateaus by encouraging a more balanced physiological state.

Seeking professional help, such as talking with a nutritionist or fitness trainer, can provide specific techniques for overcoming plateaus. These specialists may examine individual situations, identify potential hazards, and offer specific guidance to recalibrate nutrition and activity routines. Their knowledge might give a useful perspective to breaking past the weight loss plateau.

Recognizing and breaking through weight loss plateaus is a dynamic process that requires a diversified strategy. By recognizing the signs of a plateau, introducing variety into diet and exercise routines, reassessing dietary habits, incorporating HIIT and strength training, addressing stress levels, and seeking professional guidance, individuals can navigate through plateaus and continue progressing toward their weight loss goals.

Dealing with Setbacks and Staying Motivated

Dealing with setbacks and sustaining motivation are vital components of any health and wellness journey, particularly in the goal of weight management. Setbacks are unavoidable and can take different forms, from short slips in dietary choices to unforeseen life occurrences. Developing resilience and techniques to stay motivated in the face of failures is vital for long-term success.

When faced with setbacks, it's crucial to develop a proactive rather than reactive approach. Instead of concentrating on guilt or resentment, embrace setbacks as learning opportunities. Analyze the variables contributing to the setback, identify triggers, and assess how to mitigate them in the future. This strategy transforms setbacks into stepping stones for growth and improvement.

Maintaining a positive outlook during setbacks is crucial to preserving motivation. Rather than perceiving setbacks as failures, consider them as momentary detours from the broader journey. Celebrate the success accomplished thus far and focus on the opportunity to recommit to health goals. A positive mindset promotes resilience and fosters a sustainable approach to the weight management process.

Setting reasonable expectations plays a crucial part in dealing with disappointments. Acknowledge that setbacks are a typical part of any transformative journey and do not equate to a complete derailment. Establishing reasonable short-term goals gives a sense of success and keeps motivation maintained, especially during hard situations.

Cultivating a strong support system is vital for navigating setbacks. Sharing experiences with friends, family, or a health and wellness group provides emotional support and encouragement. A support system not only aids in overcoming failures but also serves as a source of motivation throughout both victories and trials.

Reigniting motivation entails examining personal goals and recognizing intrinsic sources of inspiration. Connecting with the deeper causes behind the desire for change enhances commitment. Whether it's greater health, increased energy, or enhanced overall well-being, understanding the "why" behind the journey provides depth to drive and resilience.

Implementing positive reinforcement tactics aids in keeping motivated despite setbacks. Rewarding oneself for achievements, both great and small, fosters positive behavior. This can include non-food rewards, like as a spa day or new fitness equipment, which contribute to a sense of success and help keep motivation during hard stages.

Incorporating diversity into routines can be a great motivation. Monotony can add to a sense of immobility, making losses appear more significant. Introducing new activities, whether in workout routines or meal planning, not only provides excitement but also challenges the body and mind, reigniting drive and enthusiasm for the trip.

Adopting a growth mentality is a vital element of staying motivated during setbacks. Embracing adversities as opportunities for learning and progress promotes resilience. Rather than viewing setbacks as insurmountable challenges, see them as brief detours that contribute to personal development and a more comprehensive approach to the weight loss journey.

Setbacks are an intrinsic part of the weight management path, and retaining motivation demands a proactive and positive outlook. By viewing setbacks as learning opportunities, setting realistic expectations, cultivating a strong support system, revisiting personal goals, implementing positive reinforcement, introducing variety, and adopting a growth mindset, individuals can navigate through setbacks with resilience and continue progressing toward their health and wellness objectives.

Chapter 9

Personalizing the Fat to Fit Formula

Personalizing the Fat-to-Fit Formula is a vital part of obtaining sustainable and individualized success in weight management. Recognizing that each person's path is unique, with various choices, lifestyle limits, and physiological concerns, is crucial. Tailoring the strategy to correspond with personal traits ensures a more meaningful and sustainable impact.

One crucial part of personalizing is understanding individual tastes and tendencies. This extends to dietary choices, workout habits, and even the form of motivation that resonates most successfully. Whether someone finds consolation in a particular style of workout or appreciates specific types of meals, incorporating these preferences into the Fat-to-Fit Formula promotes adherence and overall happiness.

Acknowledging the significance of lifestyle restrictions is equally vital in personalizing. Realistic goal-setting entails evaluating daily obligations, job schedules, and family responsibilities. Personalizing the formula to fit inside the boundaries of one's life ensures that the changes are manageable and sustainable. This strategy prevents the imposition of unrealistic expectations that may lead to frustration and derailment.

Understanding individual physiological responses to varied dietary and exercise methods is crucial. What works for one individual may not be equally successful for another. Factors such as metabolism, hormone balance, and genetic predispositions all play a role. By tailoring the Fat-to-Fit Formula, people can optimize tactics that correspond with their physiological makeup for more efficient and tailored results.

Incorporating a holistic approach is vital in tailoring the formula. This requires examining not only physical well-being but also mental and emotional factors. Addressing stress management, sleep quality, and mental well-being leads to a more holistic and individualized approach. Recognizing the interdependence of these factors enables a more nuanced and effective strategy.

Individualized goal-setting is a cornerstone of personalization in the Fat-to-Fit Formula. Setting precise, measurable, attainable, relevant, and time-bound (SMART) goals gives for a clear roadmap tailored to personal aspirations. These goals should represent not only desired physical accomplishments but also cover broader health and well-being objectives.

Personalizing the Fat-to-Fit Formula demands ongoing reassessment and adaptation. As circumstances, preferences, and goals alter, so too should the strategy. Flexibility is crucial in negotiating the changing nature of personal growth. Adjusting strategies based on ongoing input and experiences ensures that the formula remains aligned with individual needs and ambitions.

Personalizing the Fat-to-Fit Formula is the key to obtaining sustainable success in weight management. By understanding individual preferences, accommodating lifestyle constraints, considering physiological responses, adopting a holistic perspective, and embracing individualized goal-setting, individuals can create a formula that not only achieves physical transformation but also enhances overall well-being in a way that is uniquely tailored to their journey.

Customizing Strategies for Individual Needs

Customizing techniques for individual needs is a cornerstone in the pursuit of sustainable and successful health and wellness. Recognizing that no two individuals are identical, the customization of tactics includes modifying techniques to match personal needs, preferences, and situations. This tailored approach promotes adherence, engagement, and overall success in accomplishing health and fitness goals.

One key part of personalization is knowing and meeting varied dietary choices and constraints. Individuals may have distinct cultural, ethical, or health-related issues that influence their eating choices. Tailoring nutritional practices to correspond with these tastes guarantees that individuals are more likely to adhere to dietary programs, and develop a pleasant relationship with food.

Considering individual lifestyles and routines is another key part of customization. Strategies that effortlessly integrate into daily life are more likely to be sustained. This requires acknowledging work schedules, family commitments, and personal time limits. Customizing exercise routines and food regimens to fit within these constraints guarantees that individuals can smoothly incorporate healthy habits into their existing lifestyles.

Addressing individual fitness levels and goals is crucial in personalization. Recognizing that everyone starts from a distinct baseline enables the construction of individualized training routines. Whether an individual is a beginner or an advanced fitness fanatic, customization guarantees that the intensity, duration, and type of exercise coincide with their current capabilities and future objectives.

Incorporating tactics that reflect individual physiological characteristics further enhances personalization. Understanding elements such as metabolism, hormone balance, and genetic predispositions allows for the optimization of tactics. Tailoring food programs and exercise routines to correspond with individual responses ensures that efforts are directed toward the most effective and efficient strategies for obtaining desired goals.

Customization also entails understanding and adjusting mental and emotional aspects. Individuals may have various levels of stress, motivation, and mental resilience. Tailoring tactics to meet these factors ensures a holistic approach to health and wellness. Incorporating stress-reducing activities, motivational approaches, and mental health considerations boosts the overall success of tailored strategies.

Providing a number of options and alternatives is a significant tactic in customizing. Recognizing that individuals may have various preferences for training modalities, types of meals, or even methods of tracking progress provides for a more adaptable approach. Customization entails presenting choices that resonate with individual interests, boosting engagement and long-term adherence.

Regular reassessment and feedback are key components of the customizing process. As individuals grow on their health and wellness journeys, their requirements, preferences, and goals may alter. Customization involves a dynamic and responsive strategy that modifies techniques based on continuing feedback. This ensures that the tailored strategy remains current, effective, and connected with individual ambitions.

tailoring solutions for individual requirements is a dynamic and individualized approach to health and wellness. By understanding and accommodating diverse dietary preferences, acknowledging lifestyle constraints, considering fitness levels and goals, recognizing physiological differences, addressing mental and emotional factors, providing variety, and incorporating regular reassessment, individuals can create tailored plans that not only achieve short-term objectives but also foster lasting and meaningful changes in their overall well-being.

Adapting the Formula to Different Lifestyles

Adapting the formula to different lifestyles is a vital part of customizing health and wellness programs to the diverse requirements and habits of individuals. Recognizing that everyone leads a unique life with varied needs, schedules, and priorities is vital in designing a formula that is not only productive but also sustainable across various lifestyles.

One major factor in adjusting the formula is understanding the differences in everyday routines. Different occupations, family arrangements, and personal responsibilities result in diverse daily schedules. Customizing exercise routines and nutritional regimens to coincide with these timetables guarantees that individuals may effortlessly adopt good habits into their lives without causing unnecessary disturbance.

Understanding the level of physical activity inherent in varied lifestyles is vital in customizing exercise routines. Some individuals may have employment that involves extensive physical labor, while others may lead more sedentary lifestyles. Adapting the exercise formula requires recognizing these differences and establishing strategies that complement rather than compete with people's existing activity levels.

Adapting the formula also entails evaluating the potential impact of travel, social activities, and other rare disturbances. Strategies should be flexible enough to handle these conditions without jeopardizing overall success. Providing alternatives for on-the-go workouts, offering counsel on healthier choices in social settings, and establishing an attitude of adaptation contribute to the formula's versatility.

Addressing the varied nutritional considerations associated with different lifestyles is another key part of adaptation. Individuals with busy schedules may want fast and quick dinner options, while those with more flexibility may opt for complex cuisine. The formula should contain a range of dietary solutions that accommodate to various preferences, time limits, and cultural factors.

Considering the emotional and mental characteristics of diverse lifestyles is crucial in modifying the recipe. Stress levels, motivation, and mental resilience vary among persons with distinct lifestyles. Customizing solutions to account for these variances promotes a comprehensive approach to health and wellness. Incorporating stress-management approaches, motivational tools, and mental health considerations boosts the adaptability of the formula.

Providing options for individuals with diverse fitness preferences is a significant method of adaptation. Some may favor regimented gym routines, while others may incline towards outdoor activities or home-based exercises. Offering a variety of workout methods ensures that the formula remains entertaining and matches with various preferences, boosting adherence and long-term success.

Adapting the formula also includes acknowledging the function of social support in varied lifestyles. Some individuals may have solid support systems, while others may manage their health journeys more autonomously. Strategies should be flexible to both contexts, fostering self-sufficiency when needed and encouraging involvement with support networks when accessible.

Tailoring the formula to varied lifestyles is a dynamic and flexible approach to health and wellness. By customizing strategies to accommodate diverse schedules, recognizing the impact of varying levels of physical activity, addressing occasional disruptions, tailoring nutritional plans to individual dietary considerations, considering emotional and mental aspects, providing fitness options, and recognizing the role of social support, individuals can create a formula that seamlessly integrates with their unique lifestyles, fostering sustainable and meaningful changes in their overall well-being.

Chapter 10

Celebrating Success: Milestones and Rewards

The act of acknowledging and celebrating one's achievements is an essential component of any journey that is intended to bring about transformation, particularly in the field of health and wellness. The establishment of significant milestones and the incorporation of incentives into one's path not only serve as a powerful motivation for continuous dedication and adherence to the tactics that have been created, but they also serve as an acknowledgment of progress that has begun.

Along their journey toward wellness, individuals are provided with measurable indicators of their progress using milestones. These can take many forms, including achieving particular weight-loss objectives, becoming proficient in a new workout program, or adhering to a balanced eating plan consistently. Individuals can track their progress and feel a sense of accomplishment as they navigate through their health journey when they set clear and attainable benchmarks for themselves.

The concept of positive reinforcement is incorporated into the formula through the use of incentives as a means of commemorating the accomplishment of certain milestones. The rewards that are offered ought to be tailored to the preferences of the individual and should function as significant incentives. It is important to recognize that rewarding accomplishment contributes to a good psychological link with the journey. This can be accomplished by indulging in a soothing spa day, treating oneself to a favorite meal, or purchasing fitness gear that is highly sought after.

Celebrating achievement is not just reserved for huge milestones; appreciating modest successes is equally vital. The ability to consistently attend workouts, the adoption of improved eating habits, and the triumph over personal problems are all examples of this. People can develop a positive momentum that drives their motivation and maintains their commitment to the overall health formula when they acknowledge the incremental achievements that they have achieved.

In building a system of celebration, it is necessary to maintain a healthy balance. Rewards should be perceived as rare treats rather than frequent indulgences to prevent weakening progress. Striking this balance ensures that the act of celebrating success stays a meaningful and lasting element of the health and wellness journey.

The act of celebrating achievement extends beyond the person and can be enhanced through the support of friends, family, or a community. Sharing triumphs with others not only enhances the delight of success but also promotes a sense of camaraderie and encouragement. This collaborative celebration promotes the sense that the journey is not alone but a shared undertaking with a network of support.

Furthermore, the process of celebrating accomplishments leads to the growth of a happy mindset. By focusing on achievements, individuals shift their emphasis from the obstacles ahead to the progress made. This optimistic approach not only promotes resilience during setbacks but also creates a more joyful and gratifying experience throughout the health and wellness journey.

Celebrating success through milestones and prizes is a strategic and psychologically helpful ingredient of the health and wellness recipe. By setting achievable milestones, incorporating meaningful rewards, recognizing both major and minor victories, maintaining a healthy balance, sharing achievements with others, and cultivating a positive mindset, individuals enhance their motivation and commitment to the journey, ensuring a more gratifying and sustainable path to overall well-being.

Setting Realistic Goals

Setting realistic goals is a vital component of any successful health and wellness journey, laying the foundation for sustainable growth and long-term success. The process of goal-setting includes a delicate balance between ambition and practicality, ensuring that individuals embark on a road that is both demanding and doable.

One crucial aspect of developing realistic goals is to make them specific and quantifiable. Vague ambitions such as "losing weight" or "getting fit" lack the precision needed for effective planning and evaluation. Instead, setting concrete and verifiable targets, such as reducing a certain amount of weight or exercising for a set number of minutes per day, provides a clear roadmap for development.

Realistic goals should also be achievable within a fair timeframe. While it's natural to be ambitious, setting impossible expectations can lead to dissatisfaction and a sense of failure. Assessing individual capacities, considering lifestyle constraints, and factoring in unexpected setbacks are vital in determining what can actually be completed during a certain period.

Aligning goals with individual values and priorities boosts their relevance and meaning. Whether the focus is on increasing overall health, strengthening physical performance, or obtaining a certain aesthetic end, the goals should resonate with personal reasons. This alignment develops a deeper connection to the objectives, boosting the chance of ongoing engagement.

The concept of having short-term and long-term goals offers a systematic approach to advancement. Short-term goals operate as stepping stones, providing individuals with regular achievements that contribute to a sense of accomplishment. Long-term goals, on the other hand, provide a broader vision, directing the overall trajectory of the health and wellness journey.

In creating realistic goals, it is vital to remember the holistic nature of health. Goals should transcend just physical outcomes and embrace mental, emotional, and social dimensions. Incorporating objectives relating to stress management, sleep enhancement, or social involvement adds to a more holistic and balanced approach to well-being.

The process of goal-setting involves constant reassessment and adjustment. As individuals proceed on their health journey, factors such as changing circumstances, growing priorities, and new information may require revisions to early goals. This adaptability guarantees that the goals stay relevant and reachable throughout the changing nature of the wellness journey.

Moreover, appreciating modest wins along the way is crucial to retaining motivation and building a positive outlook. Acknowledging and praising success, no matter how modest, helps to create a sense of accomplishment and sustains the dedication to the overall health and wellness goals.

Setting realistic goals is an art that involves clarity, pragmatism, and a profound awareness of individual aspirations. By making goals specific and measurable, aligning them with personal values, considering short-term and long-term perspectives, addressing holistic well-being, adapting to changing circumstances, and celebrating successes, individuals can establish a roadmap that not only challenges them but also propels them toward sustained health and wellness.

Rewards that Reinforce Healthy Habits

Establishing and keeping healthy behaviors is a journey that can be considerably facilitated by including well-considered rewards. The concept of rewards extends beyond mere indulgences; it entails providing positive reinforcements that correspond with the aim of a better lifestyle. These rewards play a vital role in motivating, developing adherence to new behaviors, and contributing to the overall success of the health journey.

One useful technique is to add rewards that directly reinforce the established healthy habits. For instance, rewarding consistent exercise with a new pair of running shoes or training apparel not only serves as a motivational incentive but also reinforces the commitment to physical activity. Such rewards contribute to the durability of good habits by offering tools or resources that support their continuation.

Incentivizing favorable dietary choices is another key part of establishing healthy habits. Rather than relying on food-related rewards that may contradict the health path, individuals can opt for rewards that correspond with their nutritional goals. This could mean treating oneself to a cooking class to learn new healthy recipes or investing in excellent kitchen appliances to assist in the preparation of nutritious meals.

Non-material rewards that focus on mental and emotional well-being contribute greatly to reinforcing healthy habits. Activities such as a soothing spa day, a weekend getaway, or a day of leisure spent on a beloved hobby serve as important rewards. These awards highlight the importance of mental health in the whole wellness journey, emphasizing the idea that self-care is a critical component of the pursuit of a healthy lifestyle.

The concept of experiential rewards adds a dynamic and pleasurable component to the reinforcement process. Instead of material items, individuals might reward themselves with experiences that match their wellness goals. This could be a weekend hiking excursion, a health retreat, or participation in a fitness event. Experiential rewards build memorable and positive links with the pursuit of a healthier lifestyle.

Social rewards, incorporating the engagement of friends or family, can be an effective reinforcement approach. Planning activities such as group exercises, healthy cooking sessions, or outdoor trips with loved ones not only adds a social dimension to the wellness journey but also improves the support system. Positive social reinforcement adds to prolonged motivation and commitment to healthy practices.

Moreover, the idea of self-reflection and mindfulness as rewards reinforces the significance of mental and emotional balance. Incorporating practices such as meditation sessions, mindfulness retreats, or even a regular journaling routine into the incentive system encourages a holistic approach to well-being. These prizes inspire individuals to acquire a deeper awareness of themselves and their wellness journey.

Rewards that encourage healthy habits go beyond the ordinary and dig into tactics that connect with the ideals of the wellness journey. By integrating rewards that support healthy habits directly, incentivizing positive dietary choices, incorporating non-material rewards for mental and emotional well-being, embracing experiential rewards, involving social reinforcement, and emphasizing mindfulness as a reward, individuals can create a reinforcement system that not only motivates but also aligns seamlessly with their pursuit of a healthier lifestyle.

Chapter 11

Beyond Weight: Monitoring Overall Health

Monitoring general health extends beyond the typical focus on weight, providing a more holistic perspective on one's well-being. While weight is a useful statistic, a holistic approach to health requires examining many indications that collectively portray a more complex picture of an individual's physical, mental, and emotional status.

One key part of monitoring general health is paying attention to body composition. This entails analyzing the distribution of muscle, fat, and other tissues throughout the body. Understanding body composition extends beyond the numbers on a scale, allowing individuals to measure the effectiveness of their fitness and diet plans in gaining lean muscle and eliminating excess fat.

In addition to body composition, cardiovascular health is a crucial measure to monitor. Regular measurements of heart rate, blood pressure, and cholesterol levels provide insights into the efficiency of the cardiovascular system. A robust and well-functioning heart is crucial to general health, and monitoring these vital indicators helps individuals make informed decisions about their lifestyle and habits.

Regular check-ups and testing for various health markers contribute considerably to monitoring overall health. Blood tests that measure glucose levels, lipid profiles, and hormone levels provide vital information on metabolic health. Regular dental and eye examinations, as well as skin checks, help with overall health monitoring, addressing any abnormalities before they become more severe concerns.

Cognitive health is an often-overlooked factor of general well-being. Monitoring cognitive function entails testing memory, attention, and executive function. Engaging in activities that challenge the mind, such as puzzles or acquiring new abilities, can contribute to cognitive wellness. Regular mental health check-ins with professionals further strengthen one's awareness of emotional well-being.

Physical fitness tests are crucial components in monitoring overall health. These examinations go beyond weightlifting capacity or running speeds, incorporating flexibility, balance, and functional movement patterns. A well-rounded fitness profile ensures that individuals are not just strong and nimble but also capable of doing daily activities with ease.

Emotional and mental well-being are crucial to the entire health equation. Regular self-reflection, mindfulness techniques, and seeking professional treatment when needed contribute to mental health monitoring. Emotional intelligence and the ability to regulate stress are key components in sustaining a balanced and resilient mental state.

Beyond the concrete measures, measuring general health entails paying attention to how individuals feel on a day-to-day basis. Energy levels, sleep quality, and mood serve as subjective markers that provide vital insights into the effectiveness of lifestyle decisions. Tuning into these internal indicators allows individuals to make improvements to their habits proactively.

Monitoring overall health transcends a narrow focus on weight and includes a multidimensional approach. By examining body composition, cardiovascular health, regular check-ups, cognitive function, physical fitness, emotional and mental well-being, and internal cues, individuals can create a more thorough understanding of their entire health. This complete approach helps individuals to make informed decisions that prioritize not only weight management but also the holistic pursuit of a healthier and happier life.

Key Health Indicators for a Balanced Life

Balancing the various parts of life needs a comprehensive examination of crucial health indicators that extend beyond just physical well-being. These indicators offer a holistic perspective on one's total health, comprising physical, mental, emotional, and social components. By recognizing and actively monitoring these essential health indicators, individuals can build a more balanced and meaningful existence.

Physical health acts as a foundational pillar for a balanced life. Beyond weight, crucial indications include body composition, which examines the distribution of muscle and fat, and cardiovascular health, represented in measures such as heart rate, blood pressure, and cholesterol levels. Regular exercise, a decent diet, and appropriate sleep help to sustain optimal physical health, creating the groundwork for a balanced and vigorous existence.

Mental well-being is a critical factor often undervalued in the pursuit of balance. Cognitive health indicators, such as memory, attention, and executive function, provide insights into mental sharpness. Engaging in activities that excite the mind, handling stress effectively, and cultivating emotional resilience contribute to a sound mental state, crucial for navigating life's complexities.

Emotional health goes hand in hand with mental well-being, comprising the ability to understand, express, and control emotions. Key markers include emotional intelligence, self-awareness, and the capacity to cope with stress. Nurturing healthy relationships, practicing mindfulness, and getting support when required are key components of maintaining emotional balance.

Social connections and relational health are often underestimated but play a key part in creating a balanced existence. The quality of connections, both personal and professional, contributes greatly to overall well-being. Key markers in this arena include communication skills, empathy, and the ability to make meaningful connections. Cultivating a supportive social network provides a sense of belonging and enhances the tapestry of one's life.

Adequate sleep stands as a fundamental health indicator that benefits both physical and mental well-being. Quality sleep is vital for good functioning, altering mood, cognitive performance, and general resilience. Monitoring sleep habits, having a consistent sleep regimen, and providing a favorable sleep environment contribute to maintaining this key health indicator.

Financial health is an often-underestimated part of a healthy existence. Key factors include budgeting skills, financial literacy, and the ability to manage and reduce debt. Achieving financial stability and planning for the future are crucial components that lessen stress and help to a more secure and balanced living.

Personal growth and a feeling of purpose are vital to a fulfilling existence. Key signs include a dedication to continual learning, developing and attaining personal objectives, and a sense of fulfillment in one's achievements. Continual self-reflection, the pursuit of passions, and a firm knowledge of one's principles contribute to a sense of purpose that anchors and motivates individuals onward in their quest toward balance.

Balancing the multiple dimensions of life includes continuously monitoring important health indicators across physical, mental, emotional, social, and financial realms. By paying attention to these signs and making conscious decisions that match with overall well-being, individuals can cultivate a balanced and meaningful existence that goes beyond the surface and incorporates the richness of human experience.

Regular Check-ups and Health Assessments

Regular checkups and health assessments serve as vital components of proactive healthcare, providing individuals with useful insights into their well-being and enabling early detection of any health issues. Embracing a preventive approach, these frequent exams aid in the preservation of good health and the prevention of more major health concerns.

One of the key benefits of regular checks is the chance for early detection and prevention of diseases. Routine screenings, blood tests, and diagnostic evaluations undertaken during checks assist healthcare practitioners in uncovering potential health issues before they emerge into catastrophic illnesses. Timely management and lifestyle improvements can considerably minimize the advancement of such disorders, encouraging better health outcomes.

These health exams expand beyond the physical realm, embracing mental and emotional well-being. Mental health checkups and evaluations give a venue for individuals to discuss concerns linked to stress, anxiety, or mood disorders with healthcare professionals. This proactive strategy helps destigmatize mental health talks and facilitates prompt interventions, such as counseling or therapy, to improve overall emotional wellness.

Regular checkups also serve a significant role in establishing a baseline for an individual's health status. Through comprehensive examinations, healthcare practitioners can track changes in critical health indicators over time. This baseline becomes invaluable for detecting small variations that may suggest emerging health issues, driving individualized healthcare efforts, and enabling individuals to make educated decisions about their well-being.

Preventive treatment, a cornerstone of frequent health assessments, encompasses immunizations, tests, and lifestyle counseling targeted at minimizing the risk of chronic diseases. Vaccinations protect against infectious diseases, tests uncover potential health hazards, and lifestyle coaching helps individuals toward healthier habits. The fusion of these aspects permits individuals to take an active role in preventing health disorders and preserving general well-being.

Beyond disease prevention, regular checks build a proactive and collaborative relationship between individuals and their healthcare professionals. These appointments establish a forum for open discussion, where individuals can discuss their health concerns, seek advice on lifestyle improvements, and actively engage in decisions relating to their healthcare. This collaborative approach boosts healthcare participation and provides a sense of empowerment in managing one's health.

Age-appropriate health evaluations match preventive strategies to an individual's life stage. Whether it involves monitoring cholesterol levels, screening for particular cancers, or addressing age-specific health concerns, these examinations respond to the distinct needs of individuals at different periods of life. This tailored approach guarantees that healthcare solutions fit with the evolving health requirements of each individual.

Regular checks and health evaluations are the cornerstone of preventive healthcare, delivering a complete and proactive approach to well-being. From early diagnosis of potential health issues to individualized preventive care and promoting open communication between individuals and healthcare professionals, these routine exams assist considerably in preserving optimal health throughout the various stages of life. Embracing the habit of regular checkups is a proactive step toward developing a health-conscious and empowered lifestyle.

Chapter 12

Sustainable Approaches to Weight Maintenance

Sustainable approaches to weight maintenance necessitate adopting long-term tactics that prioritize general health and well-being, transcending the fleeting and usually restrictive nature of fad diets. These approaches realize that maintaining a healthy weight is a hard effort that needs a balanced integration of nutrition, physical activity, and lifestyle factors.

The cornerstone of sustainable weight maintenance is an emphasis on balanced nutrition. Rather than succumbing to severe calorie limitations or removing entire food groups, patients are encouraged to adopt a well-rounded and nutrient-dense diet. This involves integrating a mix of fruits, vegetables, lean proteins, complete grains, and healthy fats into daily meals. By embracing a broad and pleasurable dietary pattern, individuals can meet their nutritional needs while fostering a sustained and joyful connection with food.

Physical activity forms a critical part of sustained weight maintenance. Rather than depending only on intensive and sporadic fitness programs, a sustainable approach comprises finding enjoyable and consistent sorts of exercise. This could include activities like walking, cycling, swimming, or indulging in recreational sports. The goal is to develop a regimen that aligns with individual tastes and can be sustained over the long term, supporting not just weight management but overall health and fitness.

Behavioral modifications are crucial in sustainable weight maintenance. This involves establishing mindful eating habits, being cautious of portion sizes, and paying attention to hunger and fullness cues. Developing a healthy relationship with food requires knowing the emotional triggers for eating and finding different techniques to cope with stress or boredom. These behavioral alterations lead to a healthy lifestyle that supports permanent weight management.

Setting fair and achievable goals is another key aspect of sustainable weight maintenance. Rather than fixating on rapid and dramatic weight loss, individuals are taught to achieve realistic milestones. This strategy produces a sense of accomplishment and inspires individuals to continue dedicated to their long-term health aims. Celebrating these victories stimulates positive behaviors and aids in building a durable and optimistic outlook.

Support systems play a significant role in sustained weight maintenance. Building a network of encouragement, whether through friends, family, or community groups, provides vital emotional and practical support. Sharing experiences, exchanging advice, and having a solid support system can help individuals handle barriers and stay motivated on their journey toward lasting weight management.

Mindful and intuitive eating methods help substantially to sustain weight maintenance. This includes being receptive to hunger and fullness signs, loving each bite, and enjoying meals without interruptions. By establishing a thoughtful attitude to eating, individuals build a healthy relationship with food, making it simpler to maintain a balanced and sustainable weight over time.

Sustainable approaches to weight maintenance focus on long-term health and well-being over short-term treatments. By embracing balanced food, consistent physical exercise, behavioral changes, realistic goal-setting, supporting networks, and mindful eating habits, individuals can construct a lifestyle that not only supports weight control but contributes to overall health and vitality. This holistic and sustainable outlook provides a good and enduring method to maintaining a healthy weight throughout life.

Transitioning from Weight Loss to Maintenance

Transitioning from the active phase of weight loss to maintenance is a significant point in one's wellness journey. This phase needs a conscious adjustment in perspective and approach, stressing the consolidation of good behaviors formed during the weight-loss period while adapting to the intricacies of maintaining a stable weight.

A crucial factor throughout this transition is recalibrating food habits. While attention during weight loss frequently relies on calorie deficits, maintenance demands an awareness of energy balance. Individuals need to select a sustainable and realistic calorie intake that fits with their energy expenditure. This change entails a conscious approach to diet, stressing the consumption of nutrient-dense meals while incorporating occasional pleasures in moderation.

The significance of regular physical activity persists during the shift to maintenance. While the intensity and frequency may be altered, keeping an active lifestyle is vital. This could involve finding satisfaction in various forms of exercise, from cardiovascular activities to strength training, ensuring that the chosen program matches with personal preferences and can be sustained over the long term.

Behavioral changes play a vital part in effectively switching to weight maintenance. Learning to detect and respond to hunger and fullness signs becomes vital. Cultivating mindful eating habits, keeping alert to emotional triggers, and making conscientious food choices contribute to a sustainable approach. The idea is to build a healthy relationship with food that survives beyond the planned periods of weight loss.

Setting reasonable and attainable goals continues to be crucial during the transition phase. Shifting the focus from the scale to broader health markers, like exercise levels, energy levels, and overall well-being, helps individuals assess progress beyond just weight metrics. This holistic approach creates a positive mindset and reinforces the commitment to a healthy and balanced lifestyle.

The mental transition from a weight loss perspective to one of maintenance entails embracing the concept of a lifelong journey. Recognizing that maintaining a healthy weight is an ongoing process helps individuals negotiate fluctuations and problems with perseverance. This mental resilience is a vital component in successfully transitioning and sustaining the successes accomplished during the weight loss phase.

Building a comprehensive support system remains vital. While the dynamics may alter from aggressive weight loss encouragement to maintaining a healthy lifestyle, having a network of support is vital. Sharing experiences, receiving advice, and celebrating successes with friends, family, or support groups contribute to a sense of community and reaffirm the commitment to long-term health.

Transitioning from weight loss to maintenance is not just a finish but a continuance of the wellness journey. It requires fine-tuning the habits acquired during the weight reduction phase, modifying them to suit the requirements of weight maintenance, and embracing a holistic approach that stresses total health and well-being. Successful navigation of this shift rests on a balanced and sustainable integration of diet, physical activity, and mental well-being into the fabric of daily life.

Creating a Lifelong Healthy Lifestyle

Creating a lifelong healthy lifestyle is a dynamic and evolving process that extends beyond short-term goals, stressing sustainable activities that support overall well-being. At its foundation, this path entails creating habits and choices that lead to a healthy and meaningful existence, spanning physical, mental, and emotional aspects.

Central to the building of a lifetime healthy lifestyle is the cultivation of mindful eating habits. This involves paying attention to hunger and fullness signs, relishing each bite, and making deliberate food choices. By cultivating a profound connection with the act of eating, individuals can develop a lasting relationship with food that goes beyond restrictive diets and welcomes nourishment.

Regular physical activity remains a cornerstone of a lifetime healthy lifestyle. Rather than considering exercise as a temporary technique for weight loss, integrating fun and sustainable activities into everyday routines is crucial. Whether it's brisk walks, yoga sessions, or leisure sports, selecting activities that correspond with personal preferences ensures that physical activity becomes a lasting and joyful part of life.

Nutrition literacy plays a critical role in developing a lifelong healthy lifestyle. Understanding the nutritional content of different foods helps consumers to make informed decisions that support their health goals. This involves recognizing the value of a balanced diet, including a range of nutrient-dense foods, and being cautious of portion sizes.

Embracing mental well-being is vital to a lifelong healthy lifestyle. This requires not only controlling stress but also prioritizing self-care activities that promote relaxation and emotional equilibrium. Techniques such as mindfulness, meditation, and indulging in hobbies contribute to a holistic approach that nourishes mental health over the long run.

Sleep hygiene is often undervalued yet has a key role in supporting overall health. Establishing consistent sleep patterns and maintaining a suitable sleep environment are key parts of a healthy lifestyle. Quality sleep improves physical recovery, mental clarity, and emotional resilience, leading to a firm foundation for lifetime well-being.

Cultivating social ties is another part of a healthy lifestyle that extends beyond individual actions. Building and maintaining healthy relationships with friends, family, and community contribute to emotional well-being and provide important support during life's hardships. The sense of community develops a common commitment to health and well-being.

Continual learning and adaptation are crucial characteristics of people who successfully develop a lifelong healthy lifestyle. Staying educated about new breakthroughs in nutrition, exercise, and overall wellness allows individuals to refine their approaches over time. This adaptability guarantees that the chosen lifestyle stays relevant and successful in the face of altering health priorities.

Creating a lifetime healthy lifestyle is not about harsh rules or quick cures; it's about building a foundation of lasting habits that evolve with an individual's changing requirements. By embracing mindful eating, regular physical activity, nutrition literacy, mental well-being practices, quality sleep, social connections, and a commitment to continual learning, individuals can weave together a lifestyle that supports their health and vitality throughout the various chapters of life. This holistic approach transforms health into a lifelong adventure, driven by a feeling of balance, self-awareness, and a real appreciation for the richness of a healthy and satisfying life.

Chapter 13

Case Studies: Real Stories of Transformation

In investigating genuine tales of transformation through case studies, we get insights into the tangible and often inspiring paths of individuals who have undergone amazing changes in their lives. These anecdotes serve as testaments to the power of resilience, dedication, and the quest for a healthier, more satisfying existence.

One intriguing case study includes Sarah, a working professional in her thirties who decided to start on a weight loss and fitness quest. Battling the pressures of sedentary work and the availability of fast food, Sarah found herself in a position where her health was jeopardized. Through a slow but constant transformation in her lifestyle—incorporating regular exercise, making thoughtful nutritional choices, and emphasizing self-care—Sarah not only shed excess weight but also experienced enhanced energy levels and a renewed sense of confidence.

John's tale is another striking demonstration of transformation. Diagnosed with obesity-related health difficulties, John accepted the reality that his well-being was in jeopardy. With the help of healthcare professionals, he took a holistic approach to weight management. Adopting a balanced diet, engaging in regular physical activity, and treating underlying emotional causes, John not only healed his health concerns but also developed a renewed enthusiasm for life.

The journey of transformation extends beyond bodily changes, as evidenced in Emily's case. Struggling with stress and anxiety, Emily sought a comprehensive approach to well-being. Through the integration of mindfulness activities, such as meditation and yoga, into her daily routine, Emily not only achieved emotional stability but also saw beneficial adjustments in her entire health. Her tale shows the interdependence of mental and physical well-being.

These case stories show the multiplicity of paths individuals take toward transformation. From weight reduction to mental well-being, each journey is unique, reflecting the individualized nature of health and lifestyle changes. The underlying thread across these stories lies in the commitment to sustainable habits, a readiness to adapt, and the realization that transformation is an ongoing process.

Moreover, these real stories debunk the assumption of a one-size-fits-all approach. They emphasize the necessity of adapting approaches to individual needs, understanding that what works for one person may not be suitable for another. This awareness of personalization emerges as a critical aspect of the success of these transitions.

Case studies of real-life transitions serve as powerful tales that illustrate the possibilities for positive change. By sharing these experiences, we offer glimpses into the challenges, successes, and growth of individuals who have embraced the road of transformation, inspiring others to embark on their paths toward healthier and more fulfilled lives.

Inspiring Journeys from Fat to Fit

Embarking on amazing journeys from fat to fit uncovers storylines of courage, resilience, and the transformational power of the human spirit. These tales of personal successes resonate with the universal desire for positive change and serve as beacons of motivation for those on similar paths.

Meet Alex, whose path from a sedentary lifestyle to a fit and active one is a testament to the power of incremental, lasting adjustments. Faced with the constraints of a desk job and poor eating habits, Alex made small but steady efforts toward fitness. Incorporating short daily walks, opting for nutritional meals, and progressively adopting more rigorous activities, Alex not only reduced excess weight but also established a fresh enthusiasm for an active lifestyle.

Then there's Maria, a mother of three, whose amazing path challenges the belief that time restrictions are insurmountable impediments to fitness. Balancing a tight schedule, Maria discovered the transformational impact of effective exercises and diet preparation. By prioritizing self-care and adopting health-conscious choices, she not only achieved her weight reduction objectives but also became a source of inspiration for her family, building a culture of well-being inside her household.

The account of David, a retiree in his sixties, illustrates that age is not a limitation to reaching fitness goals. Battling the sedentary consequences of retirement, David committed himself to a regimen of strength training and cardiovascular activities. His narrative dispels the myth that fitness is reserved for the younger generation, illustrating that with perseverance and adaptability, anyone can achieve astonishing transformations at any age.

These amazing experiences illustrate the concept that the path to fitness is diverse and specifically customized to each individual. What links these storylines is the unflinching dedication to sustainable transformations, debunking the appeal of short cures and stressing the benefits of patient, continuous effort.

Importantly, these examples highlight the entire nature of development. Beyond physical changes, individuals often experience mental and emotional shifts, discovering renewed confidence, resilience, and a positive attitude toward life. This holistic approach to well-being underlines the concept that fitness is not simply a destination but a constant, enjoyable journey.

These amazing journeys from fat to fit expose the accomplishments of regular folks who, through determination and resilience, altered their lives. These anecdotes are not only about dropping pounds but about recovering control, embracing better lifestyles, and serving as inspirations for others to embark on their personal journeys toward well-being.

Lessons Learned from Success Stories

The success stories of individuals who have gone from obese to fit offer a wealth of excellent insights that transcend beyond the areas of physical health. These accounts provide insights into the varied facets of personal development, resilience, and the search for a balanced, meaningful life.

One significant lesson drawn from these success tales is the potential of incremental development. Many persons on these transformative journeys emphasize the necessity of gradual, sustainable changes over time. Whether it's embracing healthy eating habits or gradually increasing physical activity, these examples underline the importance of taking one step at a time and savoring the journey, not just the destination.

Another constant feature in these success tales is the importance of thinking. Individuals who have accomplished lasting change frequently share a common trait: a positive and resilient mindset. These narratives underscore the necessity of adopting a mental attitude that views problems as chances for progress, setbacks as temporary impediments, and success as a continual journey rather than a definitive destination.

The diversity of these success stories also reminds us of the benefits of tailored approaches to health and fitness. What worked for one person may not necessarily work for another, underlining the need for individualized tactics that correspond with individual preferences, lifestyles, and health concerns. This lesson invites readers to investigate and experiment in numerous ways, ultimately finding what connects with their individual needs and goals.

Furthermore, the comprehensive nature of the alterations documented in these success stories underlines the interdependence of physical, mental, and emotional well-being. Achieving fitness goals frequently goes hand in hand with enhanced self-confidence, improved mental resilience, and a heightened sense of general enjoyment. These stories highlight the enormous impact of a complete and balanced approach to health.

The importance of support systems emerges as a significant lesson from these success tales. Whether it's the encouragement of family, and friends, or the direction of professionals, having a healthy support network plays a key role in preserving motivation and managing the inevitable hurdles along the path. These narratives illustrate the significance of developing a community that fosters encouragement and accountability.

The lessons acquired from success stories in the fat-to-fit path extend beyond simply weight loss. They speak to the broader aspects of personal development, resilience, and the quest for a healthy and satisfying life. As readers engage with these anecdotes, they are urged to extract significant lessons that resonate with their objectives, building a sense of empowerment and motivation on their unique pathways to well-being.

Conclusion

In ending this check into the Fat-to-Fit Formula, it becomes obvious that the journey towards comprehensive weight management is not only about removing excess pounds but rather a transformative process that involves physical, mental, and emotional well-being. The delicate interaction of components such as nutrition, exercise, mindset, and lifestyle choices contribute to a holistic approach that encourages sustainable improvement.

Throughout these chapters, we've navigated the different components of this formula, unraveling the complexities of body composition, understanding the science behind weight loss, and delving into the crucial function of nutrition and exercise. We've investigated the complexity of metabolism, hormones, and the psychology of weight loss, generating insights that transcend standard treatments.

Crucially, the road from obese to fit is not a one-size-fits-all affair. It is a personalized voyage, requiring individuals to design strategies that correspond with their specific interests, circumstances, and objectives. Lessons derived from remarkable success stories further underline the power of incremental improvement, a positive mindset, and the need for a comprehensive support system.

As we pull the curtains on our inquiry, it's crucial to remember that the Fat-to-Fit Formula extends beyond a defined aim. It is a continuous process of personal growth, self-discovery, and the building of a sustainable, healthy lifestyle. The individuals who have embarked on this journey, as observed in real-life success stories, stand as testaments to the transformative power of commitment, resilience, and a comprehensive approach to well-being.

In the broad scheme of individual lives, the conclusion of one chapter heralds the beginning of another. The insights learned during this journey serve as tools for continued self-improvement, urging readers to embrace a lifelong commitment to health and fitness. In essence, the Fat-to-Fit Formula becomes a foundation upon which individuals may construct a balanced and meaningful existence, celebrating not just the milestones attained but the constant evolution towards a healthier, happier self.

Recap of the Fat to Fit Formula

As we ponder on the numerous features of the Fat-to-Fit Formula, a full knowledge emerges, weaving together the various elements that contribute to efficient weight management. This journey exceeds the usual conceptions of nutrition and exercise, embracing a holistic approach that incorporates body, mind, and lifestyle choices.

At the center of this approach is the realization that weight management is a multidimensional endeavor. It entails not just dropping pounds but developing a balanced and sustainable way of living. The inquiry began with an overview of the Fat to Fit journey, setting the stage for a deep dive into the important components that define our physical well-being.

Body composition, a vital aspect, was demystified to empower individuals with the knowledge to make informed choices. Understanding body fat percentage became a vital step, allowing readers to steer their weight management journey with precision. Muscle mass, frequently undervalued, takes center stage as a critical component in obtaining and maintaining a healthy weight.

Delving into the science behind weight reduction reveals the intricacy of metabolic processes and the role of hormones in controlling body weight. These insights serve as basic knowledge, helping individuals to make informed decisions regarding their health and fitness. The research subsequently expanded to the vital function of nutrition, emphasizing the need to develop a firm foundation through essential nutrients and a balanced food plan.

As we went through the chapters, the relevance of tailored methods became increasingly clear. Recognizing that there is no one-size-fits-all approach, the Fat-to-Fit Formula encourages readers to personalize solutions to their specific needs, tastes, and lifestyles. The integration of superfoods into nutrition fundamentals showed the significance of combining nutrient-rich alternatives for sustainable weight loss.

The methodology also highlighted the importance of exercise, and detailed the building of successful routines that go beyond basic calorie burning. Cardiovascular activities and strength training were emphasized as key components, each contributing to the overall objective of obtaining and maintaining a healthy weight.

Yet, the trip does not stop at the physical realm. The formula extended its reach into the psychological aspects of weight loss, emphasizing the importance of mental wellness. The psychology of weight loss, coupled with strategies for overcoming setbacks and staying motivated, emphasized the interdependence of mind and body in the goal of well-being.

Sleep and recovery strategies were studied as crucial components, acknowledging the pivotal significance of quality sleep in weight management. The formula advocated for excellent recuperation strategies, harmonizing with an active lifestyle. Beyond the immediate weight loss goals, the story broadened to emphasize the necessity of developing a foundation for lifelong health, embracing behaviors, lifestyle choices, and tailored tactics for sustained success.

In the broader scope, the Fat-to-Fit Formula transcends weight loss, delivering insights into a balanced existence. Monitoring general health, identifying important indications, and adopting frequent exams became vital to the recipe. The story expanded to incorporate not only short-term goals but a dedication to sustainable practices, going from weight loss to maintenance, and ultimately constructing a lifetime, healthy lifestyle.

Real-life success stories became testaments to the formula's efficacy, showing amazing journeys and the essential lessons learned from those who have transformed from obese to fit. The formula, in essence, becomes a tool for personal growth, resilience, and the ongoing quest for a healthier, happier self.

In the final analysis, the Fat-to-Fit Formula is more than a series of guidelines; it is a tale of empowerment. It educates individuals with the knowledge, tactics, and mindset needed to navigate their particular journeys toward comprehensive weight management. As the pages of this quest turn, they reveal not simply the wisdom of having a fit and healthy physique but the keys to unlocking a deeper, more rewarding existence.

Empowering Readers to Begin Their Journey

Now that the entire insights and tactics of the Fat-to-Fit Formula have unfolded before you, the moment has come to empower yourself to go on this revolutionary path. This is not only a book; it's a call to action to a holistic approach to wellbeing, where every step is a move toward a healthier, more vibrant existence.

As you stand at the threshold of change, remember that the journey is uniquely yours. You're not simply dropping weight; you're constructing a lifestyle that nurtures your body, mind, and spirit. The insights offered are not fixed rules but tools for you to modify into a formula that meets your specific requirements and tastes.

The path begins with understanding your body composition, accepting the science behind weight loss, and appreciating the function of muscle mass, hormones, and metabolism. Nutrition takes center stage as you develop a firm foundation, crafting a balanced meal plan that nourishes and sustains your body. The needlepoint of your transformation also includes the art of combining superfoods and establishing an effective fitness plan that suits your lifestyle.

Yet, this is not only about the physical. Mental well-being is a critical part, of acknowledging the power of your mind in molding your journey. As you navigate through hurdles, plateaus, and disappointments, remember that resilience and mental strength are vital partners on this route.

Social support and accountability build a sturdy structure, ensuring that your journey is not a lonesome one. Through inspiring stories and practical techniques, the formula becomes a living guide, offering the motivation and insights needed for sustainable success.

As you walk into this transforming experience, remember that it's not about accomplishing a fixed goal but about accepting a lifelong commitment to health. It's about enjoying triumphs, setting reasonable objectives, and acknowledging that failures are part of the process.

The Fat-to-Fit Formula is not a conclusion; it's a powerful preface to your transformation. The keys to success are in your hands, and the chapters ahead are yours to create. This is your path, and with every step, you're building a better, more resilient version of yourself. So, arm yourself with the knowledge, draw inspiration from those who have walked this path, and let your adventure begin.

www.ingramcontent.com/pod-product-compliance
Lightning Source LLC
Chambersburg PA
CBHW071204290526
45796CB00008B/138